Waking

to

Eden

Michele Morgan Doucette

ISBN# 1450586279

For Dale, Justin, and Beau
and all our ancestors.

Table of Contents

Preface

Everyone has a story in his or her bones. *Waking to Eden* is a story excavated from the bones of a woman living in rural Vermont who, while grieving a recent miscarriage, learns that she has an autoimmune disease—a hereditary condition that had been sitting dormant in her DNA, waiting to be expressed. Rather than identifying with a diagnosis of disease, she sets herself on a path of self-exploration and discovery, ultimately deciding to heal herself by changing her DNA.

From an alchemical mixture of scientific investigation, holistic healing, and direct mystical experience, a creation myth emerges in which the Garden of Eden, a template for personal and planetary health, is immediately accessible though a slight shift in perspective. The story is framed by a unique, transformational body-mind therapy known as Zero Balancing (ZB), which accesses energy in the bones of the body. The principles and practice of ZB are intricately entwined with the author's path toward healing, just like the coiled snakes climbing up the caduceus; this creates a milieu in which myth becomes reality and reality becomes myth.

Waking to Eden is the story of an ordinary woman's life—raising children, working, encountering illness, building a house—viewed from an extraordinary perspective in which cats speak from the afterlife, unborn children offer guidance, houses are alive, DNA is malleable, and human hands heal.

Everyone has a story in his or her bones. This is but one, humbly offered, in hope that sharing stories will help heal the collective human condition.

Introduction

Studying Zero Balancing can be a life-changing adventure. Once a year, Dr. Fritz Smith offers advanced ZB classes at Rio Caliente in the Primavera Valley of central Mexico. Rio Caliente is a steaming hot river running through the valley. The water is rich in rare minerals and known for its regenerative properties. The valley is a secluded and undisturbed Huichol Indian healing ground that is one mile above sea level. The land is strewn with obsidian, the black volcanic glass formed when molten rock cooled long ago. A few scattered houses, a small convent, and a church are tucked into the rolling hills. The only other development is a simple spa that offers vegetarian food, hot mineral pools, an underground steam room, bodywork, mud baths, facials, hiking, horseback riding, and lots of peace and quiet. We gather at the Spa at Rio Caliente to study ZB. It is one of Dr. Smith's favorite places to study ZB because of its clear, strong, and expansive, yet grounded, energy field.

In January 1999, I traveled to Rio Caliente for the second time to study with Dr. Smith. As I dozed in the plane, strands of my intention for the week ahead began to coalesce. An intention for a ZB session or a ZB class is a statement of the desired outcome. Having an intention clarified to the point that one is able to state it, makes it more likely to happen.

I drifted out of sleep at one point with the vision of a safety net behind my eyes. It was woven of rough rope and stiff cables that I immediately recognized as old energy patterns and subconscious beliefs. I closed my eyes and examined it, realizing that it had been there so long, it had become invisible background information. Now that I could see it, it was in my way; it was like looking through a screen. The world seemed too small suddenly from this perspective of doubt and carried the inevitability of the fall. At least part of my frame for this week of ZB: I would like to fly without a safety net.

I remembered that before leaving for the airport that morning, I picked the angel card Faith. The accompanying picture was of two angels, doing a trapeze act in midair with a very pregnant space between them. Another memory immediately tumbled into place: a bodywork session I received from my friend Barbara a week earlier. As I lay peacefully on her table, a question popped into my head.

"Who are you to take away the sins of the world?"

I remember being shocked to hear it inside the dome of my skull. "Huh? Me? I don't know. Like, who am I to be divine? Well, I'm *me*. I *am*," I said back to myself.

What a strange question. Where did that come from? I thought about the older Aramaic definition of the word *sin* from the archery term meaning "to miss the mark." So in that case, who am I *not* to do the work I have come here to do? Who am I to skip out on my duty?

I heard another voice, from my childhood. "Who do you think you are, young lady?" I started to get the feeling that I was expected to be something less than I am.   My intention was forming itself, and it had something to do with forgiving the conditioning of my youth that held me in a mentality of lack, in a place of being small and constrained, unworthy.

We landed in Guadalajara. It was my second visit to Mexico, but it was before the 9/11 World Trade Center massacre, and it was unnerving to be ushered through customs by hostile-looking men with automatic weapons. I felt like one mistake on that green customs form and it could be all over for me. But my travel companions and I did make it out of the airport alive and before we could hail a cab, one hailed us.

After forty minutes or so, with the city far behind, we abruptly turned left and passed through an arch in a stucco wall.   Suddenly, we were in a small village. Continuing along cobblestone streets in a seemingly unending maze of right angles, we might have felt uneasy if our itinerary had not encouraged us to "proceed with confidence."

The road turned to gravel at a small toll gate. The taxi driver stopped and exchanged a few words with a man who seemed to appear from the dust on the side of the road. The gate rose, and we drove into the hills on roads which jarred our brains and almost ate the taxi whole. The driver slowed to cross a tiny metal bridge over a steaming stream of mineral water. A small and simple sign indicated we were entering the Primavera Valley. Tall scrub sage grew along the road. As the steam wafted through its leaves and the desert sun dried the air, a perpetual sauna was created throughout the valley. The heady aroma was inescapable; the medicine of sage met me and crept into me.   At first it felt oppressive—like I wouldn't be able to get enough oxygen into my lungs; that feeling was probably a combination of the altitude and air saturation. It was necessary to breathe slowly and purposefully—faithfully. The extra pressure on my lungs caused my heart to lift and open, and begin to function as a breathing organ as well. Any hard edges within me began to soften. I felt vertically organized, clarified, and open.

I recognized the intoxication. I remembered how the valley seemed to amplify all possibilities. I remembered the magic of my last visit—how open my heart had become and how the spirits of the valley had assisted my journey, my learning, and my healing. Early in the class last year, Dr. Smith suggested we take time to connect with the valley and ask for what we wanted because this was a place of great possibilities. One of the things I wanted was to experience ZB from the master. I was completely captivated by the theory and practice of this work. I could think of no better way to learn it than by receiving it from its developer, here, in his favorite place to teach it. Being the archetypical caretaker, I historically do not ask for much, but the spirits of the valley were already at work. "Do it. Do it. Do it," they chanted in my ears. At a break in class, I walked up to Dr. Smith and asked for what I wanted.

He gave me a ZB session later that day and within a few hours I was experiencing an exhilarating river of energy running through me, especially through the crown of my head. I was high for the next six days. And I was still floating when I got home. I had grand insights about ZB, about the human body, and about life. My life changed in a permanent and profound way from that one session.

So, arriving here at 'Rio' one year later, expectations were high. Each faculty member was assigned to a small group of students. The groups would meet in the evenings, an informal time to ask questions, share experiences, and have tutorials. We would all receive a session from our faculty leader. I was assigned to Dr. Smith's group. Here I was again, in the power spot with the master. I had practiced enough ZB to know better than to expect a repeat of the exact same experience I'd had last year, although that's what I secretly wanted. It felt so good! I worked extra hard to find just the right intention for my session. I wanted to get the most out of my time and not miss any opportunity to grow and learn. Days went by, and I became increasingly agitated as nothing seemed to be happening. I kept listening for my intention. I wrote different ideas in my journal, but nothing had the ring of truth. There was only the image of flying without a net. I thought I had to build words around that. Finally, I realized part of the safety net was my belief that I had to be in control—that I had to "get it right." Flying without a net meant letting go of control! I had to fly with only God's arms as my safety net! There was nothing left for me to do but offer myself and my life to the service of God.

That was clear enough and certainly core enough to be a good ZB intention. But I still felt agitated. *Can I do that? Can I truly give up control of my life? What would it mean to dedicate my life to the service of God? Will I have to die and go to another realm? I do not want to leave my children motherless! Will I be called on to leave my family and live in seclusion? I want my family! Will I have to give up my life on earth? I want my life on earth!* I spent the next twenty-four hours in relative seclusion, letting my intention filter through me. I floated in the pools with my ears underwater and listened to my deepest thoughts. *What's the bottom line? I have come up against my faith. Will I entrust myself to God or not? I must. Anything less is just resistance to what is. Ah! But I can ask for what I want, too. Here it is. This is my intention: I release the safety net of old beliefs that tie me to fear and limit me. I dedicate my life to the service of God, with my family, here on earth.* That's not really control; it's just a little guidance.

I received my session toward the end of the week. It was very grounding. No huge experience—no crown chakra explosions. I took home a grounded, peaceful feeling. I was more in love with my family life than ever. I felt even closer to my husband. I had more awareness of how big a slice of the importance pie of my life was taken up by my family. I began to entertain thoughts of having another child. My sister was pregnant, and it seemed I had a run of pregnancy-related issues in my chiropractic practice. I remember thinking how it would be great to have a child later in life, so that I could experience a more conscious pregnancy, really feel the hand of the goddess in my body, and revel in that divine shaft of light for nine months. Within a month, I was pregnant. It had to have been divinely assisted because I know when I'm ovulating, and there were no regularly scheduled eggs on the road to humanity when I conceived. It was a special-forces egg on a commando mission.

Knock, Knock

August 3, 1999 was my thirty-ninth birthday. I was the mother of two young boys whom I adored and four months pregnant with my third child. The sun shone bright, clear, and bold, daring me to be alive, to be strong, and to throw my arms open in praise and my head back in laughter. But I wanted to crawl into the earth and decompose. Standing at the stove with the two boys literally pulling on my apron strings, I was experiencing some kind of radical discontinuity. Pulling, pulling, pulling, and being pushed at the same time. I was ready to burst. Something deep in my bones, away from conscious awareness was bubbling toward the sharp light of day. Some relatively normal and regular daily-mother turmoil must have resonated with this buried secret because anger simmered, boiled, and spat until I grabbed a chopping knife and whipped it toward the floor.

PWAANNGGG...

There it stood, sticking out of the yellow pine wood flooring, the ugly evidence of my anger in the light of the day.

"It's my birthday!" I screamed, not so much at the boys as at the whole universe. "You're supposed to be nice to me! You're not supposed to make me mad!"

The poor little guys didn't know what to think. Neither did I. What I would learn was that the tremendous tug and pull was birth and death wrestling with each other—in my body.

****

A problem pregnancy never occurred to me as a possibility. I had two healthy pregnancies and two easy home births. I knew how to do this. My body knew how to do this. Consequently, when I went to my first visit with Mary, my naturopath and midwife, and she could not hear a heartbeat, I was not concerned.

"It could be the position," Mary said, probably taking my lead. "Sometimes, if the placenta is low, the heartbeat is obscured. You haven't had any bleeding?"

"Well, a little spotting once, maybe twice, after sex. But nothing significant"

"Yes, well, sometimes the cervix is friable and can bleed a little after intercourse. Let's check you next week, and we'll take a listen then."

"Okay," I said confidently. If there was any fear at that time, it took the bullet train straight to my subconscious and started steaming.

Knock, knock. Anybody home?

The Brown House

Ten years ago, after graduating from chiropractic school, I moved to Vermont and started my practice in one room on the second floor of Klara Simpla, an earthy kind of general store in Wilmington. The first floor was retail space. The second and third floors held rooms for meetings, yoga classes, alternative practitioners, etc. Downstairs, they sold an eclectic mix of carefully chosen herbs and vitamins, natural toiletries and personal care items, books, groceries, Birkenstock shoes, cookware, and the most extensive selection of homeopathic remedies I have ever seen outside of a homeopath's office. The giveaway pile, an old trunk overflowing with second-hand clothes, sat at the entrance.

The store was owned and operated by Fay Hollander, a bold, independent, and purposeful woman. I met Fay when I was in Vermont to take my board exams. I had been traveling around the state with my son Justin, who was one-year-old at the time, and my sister Karen, who offered assistance and adventure. I spent a week meeting chiropractors, becoming familiar with Vermont's geography, and looking for my own personal landing pad. Two chiropractors had suggested that I go to Wilmington and meet Fay.

Wilmington is a quiet little town that sits in a small mountain valley, halfway along the forty-mile stretch between Brattleboro and Bennington, the big-town bookends of southern Vermont. We drove up the

winding mountain road to the Deerfield Valley.   I
walked into Klara Simpla, introduced myself to Paula,
Fay's daughter, and asked if I could meet her mother.
Fay lived upstairs in a one-room apartment.   Paula
disappeared into a narrow opening, and I knew by the
creak of old wooden stairs that she was ascending to the
matriarch's lair.   After a moment, she reappeared and
announced that Fay could not speak to me now, but she
would see me at 10 o'clock tomorrow morning. *Oh, I
see. One has to seek an audience with this woman.*
Well, that was intriguing and humbly expressed. I stayed
the night in town and met with her the next morning.

   I introduced myself and described my journey in
Vermont. I asked her about her history, and she told
how the store had blossomed from the days when, as a
young woman interested in living simply, she started
selling natural peanut butter out of the ski shop that had
occupied the building at that time. At the end of our
conversation, she invited me to locate my practice in her
building. She explained that she asks for ten percent of
whatever income the practitioners take in per month as
rent. There was a chiropractic treatment table in one of
the rooms that was used once a month by an older
chiropractor who came down from Springfield to treat a
few patients.   I was speechless.   I had not intended to
ask her to work there. The idea of starting my own
practice with so little overhead was arresting, and I told
her so.

   She looked into my eyes steadily and extended her
hand toward me, palm up. "Sometimes, there is an
opportunity in front of you, and all you have to do is

accept it."

So I did.

At the time, I was living in California with my husband, Dale, and our firstborn son. We had decided to move back to New England to raise our children within driving distance of their grandparents, cousins, aunts, and uncles. Dale was traveling around the world as a lighting designer on rock and roll tours. He was relocating every few days, often didn't know where he was, and had little time or perspective to decide where to relocate our lives. When Vermont called me home, he trusted my judgment. I collected a few real estate brochures when I was in the Green Mountain State, and now, back in the Golden State I set about the task of finding a rental. The first call I placed was answered by the strong, steady, and friendly voice of Scott. Yes, they did rentals. In fact, he knew of an apartment in a nice house in East Dover that happened to belong to his in-laws. We made a plan to meet when we arrived in Vermont.

The first call I placed had led to Scott. The first apartment we looked at, we took. It was next to Scott's house, and he and his family became our first friends. A few months later, when we were ready to buy a house, I was at Klara Simpla one day when Scott walked in.

"Come here, I want to show you something," he said and motioned for me to join him outside the store. "How about that one?" he said, pointing down the street to a house on the edge of the small village.

"Yeah, that's the one I want!" I agreed. "But, it's not on the market."

"The owner has been waiting for the right time, and now he's ready to sell it."

Dale and I had been driving around looking for a house that felt right for our family and would be suitable for a home office. We often drove by this unique old house, and I told Dale on several occasions that I liked it and that it would work for us. He would remind me that it did not appear to be on the market. No sign, no listing in any of the books, just a house with someone living in it.

"But that's the one I *want*," I would pout.

We looked at one other house, and then we bought that sweet house on Main Street, which has become know in our family as the *Brown House*. It was a cape style farm house built around 1840 with two later additions. It had tremendous emotional appeal. A previous owner sandblasted what was probably a century of white paint off the clapboards. They were now weathered to a soft violet gray, the color of beach stones and driftwood. The trim was the perfectly faded blue of an old pair of jeans. The house sat up on a small hill behind an old stone retaining wall which hugged the road as it curved out of town. Two rocking chairs on the large front porch kept an eye on the village. It was an elder house in town and had a respected and revered presence. Eclectic architecture inside and out gave it a timeless and intriguing air.

We loved that house. Our second son, Beau, was born there, and it was a cozy container for my children's early impressions of family life. It was also a good place to grow my practice. We were held in its charm and magic. The eccentricity within it helped us to keep moving and keep creating, but there were limitations imposed by the age and layout of the house. After six years there, and a couple of big tours for Dale, we had some money to invest in land. We bought twenty-two gorgeous acres of meadows and woods on one of the most scenic back roads in town, hoping to build a house of our own design someday. We put the Brown House on the market and began to design our new one.

Unhappy Birthday

Before my next appointment with Mary, I had a week of meals to cook, patients to care for, friends to see, and life to live. My dear friend, Julie, invited me to go out to dinner to celebrate my birthday. Julie and I wonder if we have lived and worked together in other realms on in other lives. We share a distant memory or image of moving about a village together, under the cloak of darkness, attending to some urgent need and driven by the strength of the goddess to offer assistance where we can. Perhaps we were midwives. Julie has served as midwife to many transitions in my present life. She was at the Brown House to catch Beau as he flew the coop before the regularly appointed midwife arrived. She sealed his name to his face when, as he crowned, she exclaimed, "What a beautiful face!" Beau had been our second choice for a boy's name. It became the only choice.

It was a sultry summer night when we drove the twenty miles to "the big city" of Brattleboro for my birthday dinner. The small bistro was stuffy, with the windows steamed from conversation and cooking. Stockpots clattered, grills sizzled, voices rose and fell. The tables were so close that boundaries blurred, and the whole room seemed to blend into one big, thick soup. Half of my awareness was on my conversation with Julie and half was on the other side of a misty veil, watching and waiting and trying desperately to feel my personal boundaries. And there was the additional fog of a glass of wine to celebrate a birthday, after not having consumed any alcohol in over four months. We honored our friendship between mouthfuls of pasta. As we contemplated ordering dessert, I excused myself to go to the ladies room.

Blood.

There was blood.

Too much blood.

Not spotting.

Bright, red, blood.

A rush of awareness dropped like a bowling ball into the pit of my stomach, or more likely, my uterus.

Miscarriage?

Shaking.

Fear.

In Zero Balancing we talk about the donkey and the rider as different levels of awareness in a person. The donkey is the innate, body-centered knowing, and the rider is the mind's conscious awareness. Another way of saying it is that the donkey is the body's experience, and the rider is the mind's experience; sometimes they are quite different. Well, my donkey went into a state of shock while my rider held on to her silver lining. It could be placenta previa, an abnormal position for the placenta, like Mary had said last week. *It could be a few different things*, my rider said. *Yeah, right*, said my donkey.

The tension within me had to be played out in the drama of this earthly plane, in the warm, moist container of this night and Julie's arms. Breathlessly I returned to the dining room.

"There was blood." I heard myself say.

My cheeks, which had felt rosy from the wine and from the summer sun, had drained to pale. Julie listened and watched with her midwife senses.

"So, let's not get dessert," she said evenly. "We'll get the check and go."

Walking to the car, Julie held my arm.

"I'm scared, Jewel," I began to sob.

"I know you are," she acknowledged. "We'll stop by Mary's house on the way home and see what she thinks, Okay?"

"I don't know. I don't want to bother her at night."

"She would be upset if she knew we were here and needed her, and didn't stop in."

"Okay."

****

Mary's home office was about two miles down the road toward home. We pulled into the parking area, and Julie went knocking on all the doors of the big old Victorian house until she summoned the midwife from her cozy nest. Apprised of the situation, Mary retreated to open her office, as we ascended three worn, wooden steps to her ivy-framed porch. She sat me down in a comfortable arm chair and pulled a chair up to face me, knee to knee. Julie remained standing, watching over me. By this time, I had melted into despair and was sobbing. Mary gathered information with soft, sensitive questions. I answered when I could. She was calm and objective, even though I could feel her heart resonating with mine, which was clenching and twisting. It was straining and tearing and choking and wringing out all of the blood—all of the juice of my heart. All rhythm was gone. I could see it in Mary's dark sensitive eyes— my pain, my breaking.

"I'm sorry," I cried. "It's the saddest thing I've ever felt. I'm sorry to put this on you. No one should have to feel what I'm feeling. I've been waiting to feel the quickening of the child, Mary, to feel the spirit commit. I haven't felt it."

"You don't need to apologize, Michele. It's okay to be sad. You have four months of dreams and expectations within you.

But still, she gave me the straight line. "Well, it could be placenta previa like we discussed, or you could be miscarrying. I think you should go home and get into bed and see what happens in the next twenty-four hours. If you are going to miscarry, you will start to experience cramping like labor. If you don't, we will order an ultrasound on Monday, and see what that tells us." She might have given me an herbal tincture to take home. Mostly, she gave me strength.

****

By the time we were back in the car and heading up the mountain, the amorphous fog in which I had been floating congealed into a definite bubble of shock and grief. The boundaries that had been so blurred only an hour ago in the restaurant were now acutely scribed. I was inside the bubble. Everything and everyone else was outside. Julie spoke reassuringly to me as she drove us home to our little village in the valley. Her words glided over the surface of my containment. I could hear what she was saying; her words had form and context, and I appreciated hearing them and knowing that she was out there. But I was alone in the core of this tootsie pop of shock, separated from everything else by a not-so-sweet candy-coated surface.

Julie had called Dale from Mary's office to give the family the heads up. By the time we reached my house I had stopped crying and had calmed down somewhat. Justin, ten, and Beau, five, met us at the front door. Justin looked into my eyes with love and presence, and gave me his strong, silent hug.

Beau waited his turn patiently. When I turned to him, he hugged me, his beautiful red head lying on my four-month-swollen belly. "I'm sorry the baby in your tummy died, mommy."

Beau has always been very psychically astute. Something in his five-year-old voice of truth cut through the bubble of sadness and touched my heart, momentarily comforting me. He leaned in against me, and his donkey acknowledged what my donkey knew. Innocence was the only thing that could reach through the shroud of grief.

In the same moment, however, I heard that he was making an assumption, probably because my conscious mind did not want the clarity of a dead baby in my belly. The bubble closed back up in protection, as I released his embrace. "Well, we don't know for sure if the baby is dead. We have to see how it goes in the next few days."

He didn't say another word.

In the meantime, Dale was in the kitchen, "washing the bricks." This is a family-specific term, though I would guess it's a common phenomenon, which came about at Justin's birth. We lived in a quaint little guest house on a small estate in the hills of La Habra Heights, California. Dale had been traveling on tour and was home less than twenty-four hours when I went into labor. He called the midwife, who was attending another birth (I was two weeks ahead of my due date). She assured us that these things take a while, and that she would get there as soon as she could. As I cocooned into contractions, which were getting closer and closer, Dale began to clean. I mean he got *busy*. At one point I was laboring alone on the futon, and I could hear an unfamiliar scratching outside the front door.

"Dale, what are you *doing*?" I called.

"I'm washing the front walk." He was scrubbing the brick walkway that led to our cottage with a long-handled push broom.

"Why?"

"I don't know. I've got to do *something*!"

Washing the bricks has become the term we use for any extraneous activity that burns off nervous energy.

So once again, I was retreating into isolation within my own body, and my partner, my lover, my husband was externalized. The deep physical earthquake of childbearing was a personal threshold between life and death that required focus, faith, and absolute surrender. I knew Dale was there for me even though he could not feel or know what was happening in my body. He was there for me, outside of the cocoon. He would take care of the children. He would bring me food. He would see me through whatever journey I was taking. He would watch over me—of that I was sure. Still, within the confines of my own body and my own contract with the divine, I felt alone. I was aware that Dale was having his own experience of possibly losing a child, but I could not reach out to him from the tornado within.

Labor

The claw foot bathtub we inherited with the purchase of the Brown House had become a place of refuge. The children knew if the flicker of candlelight and the scent of lavender greeted them at the bathroom door, it was Mom's quiet time.

When Mary called the next day to check on me, I took her call in my watery sanctuary. "Mary, if I am miscarrying, what's it going to be like? I mean, what's it going to look like?" I had to be prepared.

"Well," she said evenly, "The cramping will get heavier and more frequent like labor but not as intense, and then you will pass the product of conception."

"The product of conception? What will that look like?"

"It's usually a large clot of blood and tissue."

We finished our conversation, and I hung up the phone. It was all rather surreal. Twenty-four hours ago I had the next member of our family in my belly, and now some anomaly, some "product of conception" that was only fooling us into believing that it was a baby would be expelled like a science experiment gone wrong. I was being pulled along in the drama. There was nothing else I could do. I attended it with keen attention, listening, as if to Shakespeare, to the rhythm and rhyme of the action and allowing the meaning to be evoked from the author's intention across time and space. I surrendered to the great playwright in the sky.

I stayed in bed most of that day with minor

cramping but no more bleeding. Dale offered what he could in encouragement, telling me that everything would be all right. Leaning into his strength and steadiness, I dozed, wondered, and waited; riding waves of sadness, despair, and hope.

Julie came over to check on me. I was tired of lying down or perhaps impatient. I sat on the couch and talked with her awhile. We stepped out onto the back patio to take in the summer day. I laughed. How complex we are, to be able to find moments of laughter within the depths of despair.

Heaviness began to build in my belly. I think that's probably why I wanted to stand—to challenge God. *What's it going to be, God? It's already decided somewhere, isn't it? So, let's bring the story out into the objective light of the August sun.*

"I have to lie down now," I said.

Alone in my bed, Mary's words seeped into my bubble.

"Talk to the spirit of your child," she had counseled.

I truly had not heard her words until this moment. I had been communicating for months with this spirit, though not in words. It was an unformed communication, a connection from the heart. Now, at the threshold of life on earth, was the time to try language.

I spoke softly. "Spirit child, if you will experience pain or constriction or limitation that is not in your best interest, you may go. If it is not for you to be a child in our family, so be it. If you need to go, I release you. And if you want to stay in this body and be born into this lifetime with us, I will do everything I can to care for you. I will love you. I *do* love you. And you are welcome here."

The heavy hand of labor began to clamp down.

Birth

The cramping progressed into actual labor pains. Imagining a bloody "product of conception," I decided to sit on the toilet. Dale was washing more bricks and putting the boys to bed. I was grateful to be alone. After a few big contractions, my water broke and I began to pass a lot of blood. The pressure was intense, but without the searing pain of a nine-month-old head plowing through my pelvis. Beads of sweat clung to my forehead. I felt woozy. The lonely shroud of night was falling on my shoulders as I labored. It seemed strange to want to be alone and to be lonely at the same time. I felt weaker and weaker as more tissue and blood passed. My head was light, but my heart felt as heavy as lead. The contractions finally subsided, but there was still something that had not passed, still some downward pressure. The placenta?

I summoned the courage to peer between my legs, and there, hanging out of me, in the bloody toilet, was a miniature fetus still attached to our umbilical cord. I became a lioness, all instinct and innocence. Reaching down, I pulled it up by the cord, and held it in my outstretched hand. I know my heart broke when I looked on that tiny, perfectly formed little human, translucent, peaceful, and still, but I couldn't feel it. Something more basic, more instinctual was happening, perhaps below the level of emotion. I needed to finish the process. I ripped the cord with my hands. It was tougher than I thought it would be, and it was not a graceful maneuver. I was in shock. I'm surprised, and somewhat grateful, that I didn't gnaw the cord with me teeth. My head began to spin. I grabbed a towel off the rack, folded the little person in it, and laid her on the floor next to me. I called for Dale.

He entered the tiny bathroom, his eyes quickly assessing the situation. "How ya doing?" he asked sweetly.

No time for pleasantries. "It's a fully developed fetus," I announced.

"Oh, God."

"I think I'm going to pass out. I think I've lost too much blood," I slurred as I slumped over toward the floor.

I am the health care practitioner in the house. I usually handle all pressing medical needs. I became frightened now, as I realized that the patient was losing consciousness, and I couldn't evaluate her because the doctor was going into the darkness with her. *Who will take care of me?*

"Should I call Mary?" Dale asked

"Call Mary," I said simultaneously.

He must have had to page her because by the time she called back, he had called Julie and had guided me to my bed. I vaguely heard him speaking to Mary on the phone. He pressed his hand on the side of my neck. He was trying to read my pulse, but the pressure of his hand was making me feel fainter. I thrust my wrist toward him. He was frightened, too, and he fumbled with my hand not knowing what to do. This was going to take teamwork. I was barely hanging on to consciousness, knowing I had to help make some decisions.

"Time it," I said breathlessly. "Fifteen seconds. Say go and stop."

He counted out the interval on his watch. I counted my heartbeats with the fingers of one hand pressed gently on the opposite wrist. Thirteen. It felt like it took two days for me to multiply thirteen by four.

Finally: "Fifty-two. Tell her fifty-two."

Dale was staring at me and managing a little smile. "You're unbelievable," he said. He relayed the message and listened to Mary's instruction. Julie arrived as he hung up.

"She's blacking out. Mary says to put a cold cloth on her neck and make a tea out of cinnamon."

Julie quickly left to fill the order. The cold towel felt good on my neck. The sensation was a strong contrast to the pale, flaccid, sweaty amorphous blob I had become. It slowly brought my awareness back to my body. As I came to, Dale filled me in.

"She told me to find some herbs," he said. "She said 'vago vago something.'"

The diagnostician in me began to awaken. "Oh. Vasovagal syncope."

"Yeah, that. From sitting on the toilet so long."

"Okay, that's good."

What I meant, of course, was that it was better than bleeding to death.

Wrapped in Black

I was coming back—back from the brink of unconsciousness. I was crossing back to the world from Avalon. The cold compress on my neck was lifting the fog that had veiled the two worlds from each other. It was a rough landing.

Julie ascended the stairs with some kind of bizarre tea foraged from the spice cupboard and brewed at Mary's direction. A renowned herbalist, Mary probably went through a list of medicinal herbs with Dale, none of which he ever heard of, until she finally found something he recognized that would be useful to me. Was it cinnamon? Nutmeg? Oregano, maybe?

As I sipped the hot liquid, Dale recapitulated the events of the last hour to Julie. She did her fast-thinking-how-can-I-be-useful thing again.

"Where is the baby?" she asked. Would you like me to wrap him up? Is it him or her?

"I couldn't really tell," I answered. "It was so small…oh my God."

The sudden realization that I had just left the fetus, wrapped in the frayed and threadbare lime-green towel on the bathroom floor punched me in the gut.

"Ugghhh," I moaned. "In the green towel. Oooh, I think I stepped on him when I was passing out. Oh, God." The rising tide of guilt swelled in my chest. How unsacred. "How could I be so unconscious?"

"Well, Shell, you pretty much *were* unconscious," said Dale.

"Oh, yeah," I said. But what I was thinking was, *"Not good. Not good. Bad mother.*
Selfish, disconnected mother."

I turned to Julie. "In the closet there is a basket full of scarves. There is a black silk scarf, could you use that?"

And back to Dale, "Is that okay? It's the one you brought back from Japan for me."

"Yeah, sure. It's fine, hon."

Julie ventured into the dark recesses of my closet as Dale pulled up the blankets and snuggled me into bed. It was now past 11:00 P.M., and I was feeling more stable, albeit exhausted. They settled me in for the night with my dead baby, a tiny package wrapped in black silk, tucked away on the corner of the chest beside my bed.

When they left, I got up again. I walked into the bathroom to deliver the placenta, the punctuation at the end of the sentence. This is a birth, period. It is not an illness. It is not a medical event. Maybe it is not even a mistake. It's just not at all how I thought it would be.

Grief

I awoke the next day with relentless waves of resignation and guilt eroding the crystalline matrix of my bones. I was resigned to the fact that God's hand had been played, and guilty for my failure to protect the tenderness of the life within me. I knew this was bigger than me, yet I fully accepted the process of grief. It was a tricky time psychologically. Thoughts of mistakes and judgment were given enough room to air their ugliness. I shouldn't have had that glass of wine. I shouldn't have lost my temper with the kids on my birthday. I should have rested more. I should have eaten better. I should have wanted a third child more. Simultaneously, these thoughts were shoved aside by the brawn of my growing faith; faith that everything is as it should be. God is good, and everything is perpetually in order, even if I do not understand.

I was in and out of bed all day. I wanted to be alone. I collapsed even more deeply into the density of my bubble. Barely able to move my eyes to the horizon, I could not look to my right where the black bundle lay. I could not take phone calls or see friends; Julie stopped by to check on me, and I could not deny her for all she had given. She sat on my bed for a short while, but I could hardly make eye contact and apologized. Everything was collapsing inward into the black hole I had become.

****

I lay on my bed curled in a fetal position. Waves of grief crash over me. Big, tidal waves. I had never before felt such depth of sadness—utter, bottomless sadness. The black hole that is my heart disconnects me from everything else. The sadness feels like a tremendous tenderness, a loss of the potential beauty and awe that is the gift of life. I feel the loss of life like a flower closing back up before it has the experience of seeing the sun. I feel all of what life can be simultaneously with the denial of that potential. Tears are squeezed from the wringing of my heart, from my pelvis, from the earth. Everything in my world weeps for the loss of life's expression. Everything is changing. It is the longest exhale I have ever breathed.

I hear the phone ring downstairs and pray that Dale does not bring it to me. We have not spoken of phone calls or visitors. I catch a faint piece of his conversation: "Yeah. No. She's very fragile." I feel such relief. I feel understood. *Fragile* is the perfect word for what I am feeling. I feel the capacity of love for my husband expand in my heart just like the Grinch's heart, which grew ten times its normal size when he heard the Whos down in Whoville singing their Christmas song. I am not alone. He is protecting me, holding the space for me, knowing me.

I am a fragile fossil. I am brittle, old bones without flesh. If I move, I may crumble and turn to dust. I remember the mantra of Ash Wednesday in the Catholic rituals of my youth. *From dust you have come and unto dust you shall return.* The priests were right. I am returning to dust. My matrix is imploding. Birth and death are one. The tension between them is the illusion of life, and my illusion has disappeared. Time runs backward; space is negative. There is no solid ground on which to stand. But somewhere, someone knows me, and is saying that I am fragile and holding me tenderly in his heart. Someone recognizes me. He carries me, cradles me, hold my bones for me as I am being sucked out of myself.

Sucked out of my bones and sucked into the utter darkness of grief. Yet, somewhere within me, I know that through this birth and into this death is coming a new birth that will likely bring another death and then another birth—death, birth, death, birth, death, birth. It's like breathing; you breathe in, and you breathe out. You are born, and you die. It is a slow unfolding, like spring, as mother earth wakes from her winter sleep, her eyelashes rising slowly, sweeping the snow from the pine boughs, and turning the light in her eyes onto the greening fields. Each year, the earth opens new to herself. Each birth and death cycle opens me new to myself. Each morning we inhale, open the dawn of our awareness, and every evening we exhale into our dreams. We are neither the death nor the birth. We are not winter nor spring, the dreaming nor the waking, the inhale nor the exhale. We are the stillness beneath movement, the unity within the duality. We are the witness on the journey. Awareness of this place of wholeness carries me through the dark night.

What's in a Name?

The next day was torturously long. Drained of hope, I lay on my bed all day. Dale and the boys came to check on me occasionally. They innately understood I needed both solitude and support. They might leave me, lying on my back, numb and staring vacantly at the ceiling, and return in five minutes with my tea to find me curled on my side, contracting into despair, sobbing. Dale would snuggle me under my comforter for a nap only to return and find me sprawled sideways, across the bed in surrender or supplicating in yoga's child's pose.

It was late afternoon when Justin came to visit with me. I was lying idly on my back with my head and upper back propped up on pillows. He pounced on the bed, like a puppy, squatting on his knees, arms stretched out in front of him, poised to receive the grace of the goddess.

"How ya doing, Momsy?"

It was so very hard to connect. My chin quivered with the effort of communication. "I'm very sad."

"Yeah, I know." He put his head down onto the bed. "Mom, do you think we should name the baby?"

The breath flew out of my lungs. I reminded myself to reinitiate breathing.

What he is asking me to decide is whether to take it personally or not. Do we treat this as a pregnancy gone wrong, or do we invite the presence of this being that has been with us for four months into the intimate folds of our family? The options to be considered collide in my mind. To name him is very emotional. Should I risk being forever wounded with the sadness of the loss of a child? I don't know if that's a good thing. I know already that this is a spiritual event. I know it comes to me from all directions—from a place where I am whole and at one with the spirit of this child. It is a gift as well as a tragedy, and I am confused.

"I don't know. What do you think?"

"Well, it's kinda weird to keep calling it 'the baby,' don't you think?" He reduced it to simple kindness.

"Yeah," I said. "What should we name her?"

"Is it a him or a her?"

"I'm not really sure. It was hard to tell, being so small. I kind of feel like it was both. Like the baby didn't want to be only one or the other."

From his child's pose on the bed, Justin shifted gracefully, allowing a wave of inspiration to move through him. He sat up on his knees, hands on his thighs, and looked brightly into my eyes. "How about *Eden*?" he asked.

Shallow breath. Shallow breath. Shallow breath. Okay, breathe. Big breath.

"Oh, my God. That's perfect. Where did you get that? I mean, how did you think of such a perfect name?"

"I don't know. I just thought it."

"Well, I love it. Eden. Like the Garden of Eden, where Adam and Eve lived before they ate the fruit of the Tree of Knowledge. Like heaven on earth...." I trailed off into my imagination, collecting all the images, connecting all the dots: male and female unashamed, divine children living in an earthly garden, snakes, apples, knowledge, choices, and free will!

Justin indulged my inner digression for a moment. "So, Mom, is that the name?"

"Well, let's ask dad because I wouldn't want to name him without dad."

"Do you think he'll like it?"

"I think he'll like anything we decide, but it would be right to ask him."

"I'll go ask him now."

"Okay, sweetie."

The God of Cats

Spontaneous ceremony has been a part of my adult spiritual life since I had distanced myself from organized religion while in college, so it naturally became a part of my family's spiritual life.   I was raised a Catholic and followed the prescribed course of religious education and initiation from baptism at birth through confirmation at age fourteen. Discontent first surfaced when I was required to report which saint's name I had chosen for my confirmation name and why I'd chosen that saint to my parish priest. Each student in our church confirmation class was scheduled to meet, one on one, with Father Hanley for this ritual, which I thought was cool. I liked Father Hanley; he was young and had a casual air about him. He liked to make the parish laugh when he said mass. I thought I had picked the absolute best confirmation name for myself and was proud to be naming myself after a saint. I was sure to please the priest and basically, that's what I thought religious education was all about—make the priest think you're a good girl.

"So, young lady, what name have you chosen for your confirmation?"

"My confirmation name will be Christine."

"Ahh, *very* good. And why have you chosen the name Christine?"

"Well, I like Saint Christopher because he helped carry the children over the water." I went on to tell him a story about my chosen saint. By the time I was done, his face had hardened, and his body had stiffened.

"I *thought* you would have chosen Christ as your saint," he said condescendingly.

My pride melted instantaneously into shame. It seemed so obvious now, but I never considered naming myself after Christ. Wouldn't the priests have thought that presumptuous? I didn't even know the Big Guy was in the game. I thought it was just the regular saints, and anyway, Christ probably would have been very happy with my choice of St. Christopher. I tried to be good and make the priest happy. The priest did his duty and made me feel as guilty as possible for the sinner that I am.

After several more disappointments and few more cups-o-guilt, my ability to faithfully follow the church fathers disintegrated. The velvet mystery that was the holy chalice of my youth was dismantled along with the old wooden church on the main street of my hometown. Without that structure, I was open to something else, and something else found me.

After graduating from the University of Massachusetts with a degree in biochemistry, I found a job with a company that developed and manufactured medical diagnostic tests. I lived in "the upstairs" of my grandmother's house in an apartment that had been vacant since long-time residents and friends of my grandmother had died years ago. It was the summer of 1979; I had a good job, and my own place to live. My on-again/off-again boyfriend had stayed behind in Amherst, and although I was probably missing him, I totally loved my independence.

One Saturday morning, I was standing on the rooftop porch taking in the sunshine and preparing to go for a bike ride. The day was stunningly crisp and clear, and the air was warm and soft. I felt so blessed and lucky. Then I *was* blessed. Something happened that had no name. I was washed with bliss. It seemed to come from above and move over me like warm molasses. I was ecstatic for no apparent reason. It was pure happiness. My physical heart was palpable in my chest, and it was wildly excited. Orgasmic waves of fluttering, originating inside the muscle of my heart, reverberated through my body and beyond. Grace came to me in that one moment of unity. I was one with everything; my place within the whole was perfect. The feeling lasted no more than thirty seconds, and although I have carried that experience with me always, to some degree I have also been looking for it everywhere since. The knowledge of perfect unity dangled in front of me like a carrot, drawing me ever on, searching and striving to see the divine again. It had been right there with me. It wasn't somewhere far away. It was there that day on my grandmother's rooftop porch in my hometown, just for me.

Since that day, I have looked for God in nature and have understood a more personal relationship with God. I have felt no connection to and little desire for a religious organization. I fashion my own rituals and ceremonies spontaneously from found objects and inspired words. As a family, we celebrate the major Christian holidays, as well as significant days in the pagan calendar. I love to make correlations for myself and my children between the return of the sun at the winter solstice and the birth of the son at Christmas, and between the rebirth of the green foliage at the spring equinox and the rebirth of the Savior at Easter. It seems that if we move just a little away from form, dogma, and predetermined ritual and pay attention to what is happening in the moment, then the sacred can come to us, and we can allow our rituals and prayers to arise spontaneously from within our creative hearts.

When we lived in the Brown House, we had twin black and white cats, Katmandu and Kitaro. One day Katmandu disappeared the way cats do when you live in a place where there are more trees than people. Maybe he went for a walk, found a mate, and had to stay to be the daddy, we told the boys. Maybe he met a fisher cat or a fox or an owl or a car we thought. We would call for him when we hiked up in the woods. There was always at least the hope he would return. He never did. About a year later, his brother Kitaro was missing after three days of heavy rain. We called around; we looked across the street by the river and up and down the road. Sometime during the third night, the rain let up, and in the morning Dale went over by the river to look again. Unfortunately, this time he found the cat, stiff, wet, and lifeless on the river bank. We quickly decided we had better bury him sooner rather than later. The rain had ceased, but more thunderstorms were forecast for the afternoon. The boys were notified of the discovery and the plan to go to the land and bury our pet. Solemnly, they helped collect a box and shovel, but the real emotion began to pour forth when Justin sat in the back of the car holding the box with elongated, stiffened cat legs sticking out the top. He began to weep.

"I just can't stand seeing him this way, all hard and dead," he cried.

Witnessing my son's first close glance at death, I began to cry. "I know, sweetie. It's hard, isn't it?"

And then, as if the sky couldn't hold back its own sorrow, another downpour began.

The plot of land we purchased several years ago held our hopes of building our own house eventually. While the Brown House was on the market, we spent a lot of time watching, listening, camping, dreaming, planning, and playing on that land. We held it tenderly and wove it into our future.

We brought our dead kitty to the land, and Dale began to dig a hole. Water filled it in almost as fast as he could dig; it was a muddy mess. I kept the boys busy finding a few big rocks for a head stone arrangement. The rain was getting steadily heavier. Thunder rumbled in the distance. Dale dug faster. Tears and raindrops fell into the hole until, finally, it was deep enough; we placed the cat in his watery grave. It seemed less than dignified to put our beloved pet in a puddle of brown water, but by now it was pouring, so we quickly covered him with soil and stone. What words, now, to bring peace?

I began, "Thank you, Kitaro, for being such a good pet to us. We know that you will be happy in heaven."

Through his tears, Justin added, "We know your spirit is in heaven now. We miss you, but it's okay. Maybe you'll come back to us in your next life. Rest in peace."

Dale was still catching his breath from furious digging, and I don't think Beau understood death yet, so they witnessed the impromptu ceremony silently. The rain shower passed as quickly as it had come on, and the sky began to lighten. We stood quietly by the grave, trying to feel if our ceremony was over.

One final thought came to me. "And maybe, if Katmandu is in heaven, you are happy to be with your brother again."

No sooner than the words had been given voice, the clouds parted and beams of sunlight flooded the meadow. I instinctively spun around to the east. The familiar fragrance of wet air being warmed by sunshine often portends a rainbow.

"Look! A rainbow! It's Kitaro! He's in heaven!"

All of the frowns immediately turned to smile as we gazed at this soft and brilliant stroke of God's hand across the sky. Then another smile appeared. There, just above the first, shyly emerged a second rainbow.

I gasped. "And Katmandu! They're in heaven! They're together!" We had spoken our beliefs and God said, "Yes."

My leaping heart propelled me out into the center of the meadow. The boys ran after me, whooping, hollering, and laughing. We danced around praising the rainbows and the miracle of heaven. I turned back to find my husband's eyes. I think as humans we long to share the magic of life by seeing it reflected in each other's eyes. His were laughing, too, as he walked toward us, hands in the pockets of his dirty jeans, a smile on his face, and shaking his head from side to side.

Burying the Bones

There was little discussion about what to do with the tiny lifeless form of Eden. As I rearranged myself on my bed, flopping from one position to another, lost in the arrest and annihilation of constant sorrow, Dale retreated to his shop. From pieces of scrap wood, he carefully fashioned a small and simple rectangular box. We would bury Eden in the earth with love and intention.

Purpose lifted me out of bed. I commenced treasure hunting around the house for tokens, trinkets, and talismans. How to make it sacred? How to make it real and authentic? The experience of Eden's birth/death was a deep reminder that the sacred *is* life. Life is sacred. Love is sacred. *We'll just use the stuff of our lives and our love to mark the tender presence of Eden.* I collected shells, rocks, and feathers from shelves and window sills. Explaining to the boys that we were going to bury Eden on the land, I suggested that they, too, might want to find something to offer.

We laid Eden in the little wooden box, still wrapped in the black silk scarf, and drove slowly in our black Ford Explorer to the land. The boys sat quietly in the back seat clutching their gifts in sweaty fists. Dale and I were in front with the tiny box weighing heavily between us. We didn't have a formal plan, so when we arrived at the land, we simply wandered into the woods and came to a lovely spot under some saplings, near the stream. Shimmering with dappled sunlight in all seasons, it is a place that is both alone and alive.

Dale dug a deep grave while the rest of us collected rocks. We didn't have to explain it to the boys this time. They had learned about burial from the cat. When the hole was deep and wide enough, we gathered around it.

"Should I put her in now?" I looked at Dale for guidance.

"I guess so," he said.

"But, can't we see him, Mom?" Beau pleaded.

Once again, my breath was suspended someplace between worlds. "Oh, I don't know, honey. It might make you feel very sad." I paused, took a breath, and quickly considered how much to say. "I looked at him this morning," I continued slowly. "And his skin is already getting dry and wrinkled. He doesn't look the same as when he was born. I just don't know if it's a good idea to look at him now."

"But we *want* to see him. *Please*, Mom!" said Justin.

"Yeah, we want to *see* him. It will be all right, Mom."

Another quick decision; something told me to give them this experience. Perhaps it was Eden, the third child, chiming in. I unfolded the silk scarf and held Eden where we could all look at him together. Silent tears began to flow. I wrapped him back up and put him in the box with some crystals—a clear quartz, a rose quartz, and an amethyst.

Words came from wherever they do; words of understanding and acceptance, some of which I needed to hear for myself and some for the children. "Eden, we understand that you will not be a baby in our family, yet you are a spirit that is with us forever. We release you and accept you as this body goes back into the earth. Thank you for what you brought to us and please help us to remember to listen to you always. We love you."

Dale laid an owl feather on top of the black silk and, with tears streaming down his face, spoke three words that broke my heart all over again. "Fly, little one."

Justin also offered his tears, one of his quartz crystals, and squeaked out, "Rest in peace."

Beau uncurled his fist to reveal a little green plastic figurine of an alien he found in the dust under his bed and a penny. "I thought you would like these," he said.

A Matter of Perspective

With the help of friends and family, I came through the heaviness in a few days. Denise, my office manager and good friend, slipped in and out of the house and office, seamlessly and humbly filling any need that opened before her. She rescheduled patients, sorted mail, had tea with the boys, comforted Dale, and probably cleaned my refrigerator, if I know her. Graceful Marietta quietly left a basket with a beautiful picnic dinner for us: poached salmon with dill, roasted red potatoes with rosemary, blueberry biscuits, a fresh garden salad, and a bottle of Chardonnay. Dale, the boys, and I sat on the secluded back patio, wrapped in the ripe fullness of summer trees and flowers and enjoyed our meal with a lightness that I hadn't known in several days. Julie stopped in to visit, and we shared our fairy-tale picnic with her. I felt like I was taking communion, like I was eating the Holy Communion wafer, the body of Christ. The food was prepared with love and compassion, so as we took it in, we received its medicine, its blessing.

It gave me some peace in the days following the birth that I had spoken with the spirit of Eden before delivering. I had released control and asked this spirit to move according to her highest purpose. To surrender and give space to a higher power, invites the greater wheels of life to spin; the wheels are always spinning anyway but are often too big to perceive at any given moment. This perspective of surrender was greatly influenced by my time studying Zero Balancing in

Mexico. I had been opened to the infinitely beneficent energy field of the universe in that first ZB session with Dr. Smith. The first year studying in Mexico gave me the opportunity to move beyond fear and the second year reinforced faith as a living principle; if I really experience a beneficent higher power, there is nothing left to ask for. I had to simply surrender to the will of God, and all would be well. I learned to fly without a net—to feel the fear and let go anyway. I learned to let God hold me. I learned to trust my life and keep my eyes focused with faith. I learned it all through my bones, although it would take the events of the next few years to bring this teaching to full conscious awareness.

I moved slowly through the thick, soaking grief, and as the enveloping mist that had surrounded me began to lift, I felt clarified and comforted. I reemerged into the world as if I were slowly opening my eyes for the first time. The tornado of emotion was still whirling, but it was magically softened by the containment offered by the world, as if the universe was watching me and reflecting my changing inner world.

****

We all create our own stories through the direction of our awareness—by how we choose to perceive the events of our lives. This morning, as I write, my world is quiet, peaceful, and beautiful. This morning, I exist in a warm house, looking out on the greening earth emerging from beneath the winter snow. With the first stirring of the new day, birds pour into the field. Robins hop and stutter independently. A flock of starlings alights here and there like a street gang showing its colors. A pair of goldfinches buzzes the deck. Swallows flutter and soar. Red-winged blackbirds chatter, and a lone flicker tugs worms from the mud. Mist rises from the lake in the distance and, as the dawn unfolds, I can see that the forest has begun to birth its spring color. Where all once looked gray, are now subtle shades of pink, crimson, and celadon. Beau sleepily stumbles out of the bathroom in his boxer shorts. "Whoa!" he says as he catches a glimpse of the view.

There is a pause as he walks to the wall of glass that is the south side of our living area. In the pause, I anxiously anticipate his perception, his wisdom, like a devotee waiting for the word of her guru. What will he think of the infiltration of birds?

He stands quietly observing the scene for a moment and then proclaims, "The snow really melted last night. Ice age -- over!" He turns on his heels and heads back to his bedroom.

I see the birth of spring. He sees the death of winter. It's all a matter of perspective. I may see a mystical morning and the magical migration of life, my son may see a glacial retreat, and still another may see a day destined to rain or a muddy field. I may see this birth as the traumatic yet miraculous beginning of a tale of divine inspiration, guidance, and assurance; another may see it as a bloody tragedy, a mistake, a crime.

Humarock

Once outside the veil of trauma, I had to keep moving.
The physical pregnancy may have been over, but the
pregnant voyage had just begun. I craved movement. I
needed a segue to the rest of my life. I felt restless. The
Saturday after I miscarried, Dale and I sat on the couch,
and he listened as I tried to find my way to comfort.

"What can I do for you, Shell?" he asked.
He would have given my anything at that point in our
journey together; he really loves me. I knew that finding
a way to help me through my pain would help him
through his. It seems that life is just what it is for Dale.
He's a regular guy. For me, it's a magical mystery tour,
a psychedelic dance, always swirling and shape-shifting.
Maybe that's why he looks like he is rolling his eyes at
me half of the time; he's probably just trying to gain
perspective of my ever-changing landscape. Right?

I craved the only thing big enough to quench the
searing fire of life and the scorched smell of death that
surrounded me: the ocean. At this time of rebirth, I was
reminded of my natal chart. I am Leo with Scorpio
rising. An astrologer once told me this means that it is
my challenge to express my fiery Leo nature through
Scorpio's veil of water. Sure enough, now that I had
crashed and burned, I wanted water all around me.
Through the window I watched rainwater drip from the
porch roof. The ocean was calling me from one hundred
and fifty miles east, but I resisted asking Dale to drive
me and two young boys six hours to the ocean and back

on a stormy day. I just sat there looking at him.

"What is it?" He asked.

"I really feel like being at the ocean but it's not a good day for it," I said.

"Let's go," he answered.

We piled into the car and headed in the general direction of the Atlantic Ocean.   Dale had spent many summers in his childhood at his family's cottage on Humarock Beach in Massachusetts, so he set a course for *home*, and we were there in no time.

****

I, too, had spent some time at Humarock Beach in my youth.   It was one of the closest beaches to my hometown.   My high school friends and I would sometimes drive the hour or so to the shore for a day in the sun and waves.   Once or twice I drove there by myself; growing up in a large family, I loved the independence my driver's license gave me and would seek days of solitude.

Now, as we drove to the shore together, with our family and our history in tow, I dozed off and on in the front passengers' seat. Images of the beach from twenty years ago drifted through my awareness. I wondered if Dale and I could have met there once. The scene was vivid. Was it a dream or my memory?

The day is overcast and a warm, gentle breeze is blowing onshore. A young man stands at the water's edge casting his fishing line into the surf. His heart has

*been broken by his high school sweetheart and with
each snap of the wrist, he casts away anger and hopes to
reel in something big and alive. Behind him walks a
woman in a turquoise bikini. He takes no notice of her
or she of him. He is absorbed in the rhythmic
meditation of the ebb and flow, the give and take, the
pain and pleasure of life and love. The woman stops
occasionally, slowly reaching down to collect shells and
rocks. She is fascinated by their beauty and natural
perfection. She also has a broken heart. She thinks love
and life can be like these seaside gems—free and
natural. They offer hope, and she wants to take them all
home with her. Her eyes light on a perfect heart-shaped
rock, and her own heart swells in a spontaneous moment
of bliss. She bends down to pick it up, and as she stands
back up, she catches a brief glance from the man fishing
on shore. Their eyes meet for a fleeting second before
he turns to cast his line once again into the waves. She
continues her sandy search for perfection, unaware that
she need look no further…*

****

I awoke to the familiar smell of saltwater and tidal
marshes. It was as cloudy at the shore as it had been in
the mountains, but the rain was intermittent, more a mist
than a shower. We drove past Dale's childhood summer
home, which had been destroyed a few times by the sea,
and finally by a new owner who, knowing the quaint old
cottage would never withstand another pounding, had
replaced it with a more modern home. Up ahead the

road ended at a Coast Guard compound. The gate was open and unattended, so we drove through and parked the car in a sandy lot. I didn't understand the nature of such a place, it seemed almost military, and I feared some official-looking person rejecting us, telling us we did not have the proper clearance. Dale assured me it would be all right.

The beach comes to a point there, where a channel meets the sea. We walked around the point to the right. The water was rough, noisy, and wild. The air was heavy with moisture spraying up from the ocean and down from the clouds. It was one of those days when my hair gets four inches shorter from the curls maximally contracting in excitement, like a little girl getting ready to jump into water with elbows, fists, and teeth all clenched.

Dale fished. Old buoys and pieces of rope offered themselves up as mysteries of the sea, and the boys were off on a treasure hunt. The water was too rough and the air too cold for them to want to swim. I wandered, collecting rocks. Déjà vu.

Tumbled by the tides for years, Humarock Beach is covered with smooth, rounded rocks of various sizes and colors. It is a rock collector's paradise. Maroon, mauve, dusky green, slate blue, white, black, salmon pink, amber, sandy beige, and every shade of gray. Some are solid colors, and many have inclusions of quartz stripes or swirls. Curiously, the symbols of Xs and Os are predominant markings, as if the rushing waves embraced each stone and purposefully planted a kiss or circled it with a hug before tossing it back on the shore and running away again.

The constant shuffling of rocks caused such a clatter that all other voices had to compete with it. I didn't mind; the ocean met me completely. I could see, smell, taste, hear, and feel her. She cradled me in her rocking arms. I rested there in the chaos of it all, loving the assault. We stayed for hours wandering here and there between the ocean and the channel. After picking up and listening to countless stones, I found a large oval one that was notched on one side and had a galactic swirl pattern in its belly. Holding it lengthwise in my palm, it looked like a veiled woman whose hands were raised in prayer position, as she cradled the universe in her womb. The stone offered itself as a symbolic structure in which to carry the spirit of Eden, as her bones turned to dust in the earth.

We stayed at the beach until each one of us had our fill, and then we packed our booty, along with our salty-sticky windblown bodies, back in to the mother ship and went scavenging the land for fried clams.

The State of Maine

Some friends you have for a short time, and some friends you have forever. I met Nancy when she was practicing massage therapy in Vermont. We didn't know each other long; she saw clients in my office for a few short months before she moved to the coast of Maine. We shared an immediate and natural connection—a connection that went right to the bone. We write to each other occasionally and we see each other only every few years. We do not know each other's extended family or favorite color. We have a vague memory of each other's personal history. Our personalities are dissimilar. Beneath the circumstances of daily life, we are tethered to each other. We love each other's feminine strength and honor each other's journey toward truth. When Eden kept calling me back to the ocean, I called Nancy.

She knew the moment she answered the phone that I needed her. I knew, in that same moment that she was completely present for me. The story of Eden's birth and death tumbled out in a few teary sentences.

"I need some time by myself to reflect, and the ocean is not done with me," I said as I collected myself. "I keep seeing myself in that cove by your house, and I wondered if it would be possible to stay with you for a few days."

"Absolutely," she answered automatically. After a short pause she added, "But my goddaughter will be visiting this weekend. The following weekend would be better. Would that be alright with you?"

"Yeah, sure, that's okay. Thanks. I'll call you next week."

She called back that evening and told me to come. She had digested the situation, felt her own balance, listened for the truth, and found that she wanted to open her home to me and my healing. There was no urgency to my request; it was just what had to be done, and the sooner I could heed the call, the sooner I could move on. Somehow she knew.

****

The State of Maine was a massive anaconda, swallowing me up in waves of peristaltic contractions once I passed through the steely jaws of the Piscataqua Bridge on Interstate 95. The road behind me constricted with thick ripples of concentric muscle as I was enveloped deeper into the belly of my journey. At another time I might have felt suffocated but not now. This was the right snake at the right time, and I surrendered to the inevitable transmutation. I was exhilarated as I slid through her dark body. Eat me! Digest me! Annihilate me!

My car seemed to find its own way from the interstate to Route 1 on this one-way alimentary tract. By mid-afternoon, I found myself at a farm stand just outside Thomaston. I bought bread, cheese, and apples. Continuing on, the landscape was soft and rolling, and the air, salty and buoyant. Time flowed like molasses. The ocean winked and flirted as my eyes caught quick kisses of endless rocky coves secreted between lush evergreens. I slid through the sleepy village of Tenant's Harbor and turned quietly into Nancy's driveway. Her old gray Saab with its few thoughtful decals and stickers waited graciously there to assure me I was in the right place.

Unfolding myself from the car seat, I stretched and headed down the garden stepping stones, through a driftwood arbor, to the softly weathered cape. I felt like I was in a chick-flick when Nancy emerged from her front door with a cat on her heels. Sunlight illuminated her face, and her steady eyes met mine with presence and kindness. She had a few more years of life under her bonnet than I. It had been several years since I had last seen her and she looked older than I expected. It was the kind of older that I wanted to become. She held the fullness of her soul with obvious comfort and not a trace of striving to be something else. I was instantly grateful and realized that I had sought the energy of this beautiful and grounded woman because she would witness me and help me witness myself. She would not pour emotion on to me; she would not smother me or dote on me. She would live with me for a few days. She would watch and listen, and let my discovery unfold. And I had no doubt that she would love the depth of whatever was there to be seen in me.

We toured the house, inside and out, meeting more cats, gardens, and berry patches. Gifts from the sea adorned her home. Stones worn smooth and round, driftwood, and sea urchin shells were exquisitely placed, honoring decks, gardens, windowsills, and walls.

Nancy's home smelled of nature: salt, wood, herbs, and bread.

After taking my bags up to the guest room, we settled deeper into our stories at the kitchen table with tea and homemade scones. I filled Nancy in on the details of Eden's birth, along with my perspective of the bigger picture. She listened with her ears and with her eyes. I could see her watching my face as I spoke, reading the whole story. She offered her observations, thoughts, and experiences, leaning into my truth with her own. Telling me of her own deep listening to life, she spoke of what called her out into her longing, putting aside the security of her massage therapy practice to be the artist, painting and studying with other women artists.

In the morning I awoke with the clean canvas of a new day in front of me. What colors and shapes would be splashed there today for my soul to play with? Inspired to let the creation come from listening, I reached down beside the bed and pulled the pouch of rune stones from my overnight bag. As I juggled the flat, oval stones within their gray velour bag, I realized there was not even a question to ask. Whatever guidance there was for me would emerge from the field of all possibilities. My fingers searched among the cool porcelain discs until one stayed put between my thumb and forefinger. I pulled it out and gazed at the lines etched on it; they looked like two Xs standing on top of each other. I opened *The Book of Runes* by Ralph H. Blum and looked up the symbol in the index: Fertility. It spoke of completion, resolution, new beginnings, about emerging from a closed chrysalis state, a release from tension and uncertainty, and breaking free from old cultural or behavioral patterns. It counseled grounding in preparation to open to the will of heaven.[1] I got the eerie but comfortable feeling that I was being watched over, guided, and acknowledged.

After a light breakfast with Nancy, she set off to town for a day with her goddaughter. I gathered my journal, runes, medicine cards, blanket, water, and snacks and set off on a little trail through the woods to the seashore. On the way, a small snake squiggled across the path in from of my feet. *It's amazing how the world keeps on giving.* Snake medicine: transmutation, shedding the old skin, sloughing off an old belief for a new one, changing poison into food, and alchemy. I suddenly saw this morning's rune in a new light. If you soften the angular markings on the rune, you would have what looks like two snakes coiling around each other— the classic symbol of healing, and the imagery of the Indian yogic kundalini energy rising from base to crown, creating a channel for transmutation between humanity's animal and spiritual natures. I noted the absence of my body's reflexive shiver at the sight of the slithering reptile. The shift was in process. The whole world was saying yes. Yes, you are on a mythical journey of recreating yourself. And yes, you are on a path of healing. Maine was holding me like a blue mussel, opening and closing with tides of awareness. It was opening me to insight and possibilities, and closing around me like a mother's arms.

The trail ended at a stone dune. Millions of densely

colored, smooth, round stones pushed up by relentless waves of seawater. As I stepped up onto the mound, the stones, which were packed tightly together like grains of sand, gave way to each other with a cascade of sharp and finite clacks. Sand would have hushed me, "Sshhhhh." But "shhhh" was my past: constrained, dampened, and minimized. The stones on the coast of Maine were here and now: big and loud, dense and bold, clear and present, and left no question. Stones shifted underfoot with the sound of purpose, the ring of truth, and I thrilled at the assault on my senses. I wanted the ocean to crash me down on to the rocks and tumble me smooth. I wanted all the broken places in me to be smashed by the forces of nature. If those places were to be broken, I wanted them annihilated, blasted, blown up, turned to dust, so that I could be whole again. *I am more than the sum of my pieces.* In that moment, I began to understand the rise of violence in our culture. Much of humanity, I think, is savagely thirsty for the experience of wholeness.

I looked around the beach. Slick seaweed-strewn ledges protruded from a tidal pool to the left. To the right was a driftwood museum of fanciful sculptures that the sea had carved from giant limbs and whole trees. Beyond that, a sandy crescent—a happy smile of beach created by the perpetual pounding of the waves. That was the place for me. After spreading out my blanket, I settled in and sat listening to the waves and gulls. The sky was gray, but the wind was still warm, and I was comfortable in my shorts and sweatshirt. I began my usual divination ritual by shuffling my deck of animal

medicine cards three times and choosing the card that
ended up on top. Today, the medicine that offered itself
to me was eagle. I opened the companion book *Medicine
Cards* by Jaimie Sams and David Carson.[2] Eagle
medicine is the ability to live in the realm of spirit and
remain connected and balanced with earth. It is earned
through a trial of trusting the connection to Great Spirit,
usually through an initiation that results in the taking of
one's power. *Yeah, I've been there.*

Something tickled my leg, and I looked down to
see many tiny beach spiders enjoying my blanket with
me. My immediate response was to see the problem, the
intrusion. There were lots of them, and they weren't
going away with a few brushes of my hand. Were they
going to mess up my canvas? *No, they are my painting
instructors.* I knew that spider medicine had to do with
the alphabet and was offering the suggestion to look at
the emergence of my new reality through the written
word. I did not feel the need to know more. Spider was
telling me to write.

I opened my journal, put pen to paper, and not
knowing what I would write, wrote the obvious:

*My third child was born on August 9, 1999 at 10:50 P.M.
Eden was only four and one-half months old and never
really came in to that perfect little body. Yet, we both
know that it's okay. It's all right. There is different
reason.*

The air was heavy with moisture. The first
raindrops were squeezed from the atmosphere and fell

on to the page, smudging the words *both, there,* and *reason.* The world was weeping, silent tears falling from its saturated heart. Everything in nature, including me, was so alive and so present. Each action, as infinitesimal as a thought, elicited a response from the world around me. *How can I doubt the guidance I receive in this unraveling story? How can it not be right when it all fits together better than anything I've ever experienced in the less imaginative, exclusively structural world of "ordinary reality?"*

I had cried so many tears already: tears of the mother in me, tears of the child in me, and tears for all the sorrows in life that I was not able or not allowed to cry for until now. Was Eden washing me clean of these sorrows and sins? Was I craving the ocean because somehow I knew that its osmotic nature would pull my salty tears and all the personal history they carried out of my cells? A gull called out to me. I watched her soar. I knew that she wanted me to see how easy it could be not to work hard beating awkward wings, but simply to raise them and let the winds of heaven lift me up. A devout Christian friend once told me that there was a dove that flew down from the sky as a sign when John baptized Jesus. I had missed that part of the story the first time around—the part about the world responding.

I spent the whole day being rocked by beauty. I lay in the sun when it shook the clouds off. I collected beach stones, driftwood, and sea urchin shells. When the tide receded, I walked out on the ragged rocks and let the colors, smells, and the tastes of the marriage between sea and land saturate me. I swam for long distances under the cold water. How right it felt to be in the ocean! I became my primordial self—some combination of squid, dolphin, and mermaid. Long strands of kelp danced around my face as a singular powerful tail propelled me through water that caressed every inch of my electric skin. Miles out to sea, countless aquatic creatures stirred and registered my presence. I belonged to the sea. I was home. God was baptizing me, and it was happening in four dimensions of Technicolor. When I emerged from the brine, my heart pounding with exhilaration, I felt like Dorothy when she emerged from her black-and-white house into the colorful world of Oz. *"Toto, I've a feeling we're not in Kansas anymore."*

Returning to my blanket, I opened my journal again:

I am touched by the hand of God. The spirit of the child is the gift giver. May all of the love that I could have given to Eden go as deep into the earth and as far into eternity as the love I have for my other two children. If this is why this spirit has come to me, to set this love free from within me, to shine it forth onto earth, to be the divine child of God, then I will love and honor this duty with the tenacity and ferocity with which I love and honor the duty of being a mother. For this, I can trust deeper. For this, I can be fuller.

Not another person came to this isolated cove all day until around five o'clock in the afternoon. I looked up from writing to see Nancy's partner, David strolling down the shore toward me. I finished my sentence as he approached, then closed my journal and greeted him with a smile.

"Hi," he said quietly.

I scooted over on my blanket and patted it down, inviting him to sit with me. He smiled sweetly and accepted the invitation. We sat in a comfortable silence for a while, looking out over the ocean.

"I've had a beautiful day listening to this cove," I told him.

David is a quiet, grounded man with a soft but piercing intensity. I had the pleasure of his company only a handful of times, and never one-on -one. His eyes are kind. He engenders trust and elicits truth. I knew that Nancy had not had the opportunity to tell him my story. I gave him the bones of my experience, the distilled poetry of my truth, without a lot of flowery explanation or digression.

"I was pregnant and lost the baby at a little over four months. I miscarried at home. It was like a birth and a death at the same time. It was the saddest thing that ever happened to me. It tore me apart, but it's also a gift. The spirit of the child knew it wasn't to be a babe in arms but was to be my teacher and help me to rebirth myself. I'm just beginning to understand that something is spinning me around and bringing me through a transformation. The ocean keeps calling me. Dale and the boys took me to the coast of Massachusetts, and that was really great. When it called me again, I called Nancy. I'm really grateful to be able to be here to listen and to learn and to integrate. Thank you so much for opening your home to me."

That's all it took. We were connected. He appreciated and understood me with very little effort and very few words. He approached with respect and was present with me.

After we mused a bit about life and reality, he said, "Well, I'm going to go back to the house. We'll have dinner whenever you are ready to come back."

He left as gracefully as he had arrived. This is how it can be, I thought. Humans can connect and treat each other with gentle hearts and with compassion. My heart had been broken open, and I could feel more of everything. Warm waves of vibration emanated from behind my sternum. I was ready to rejoin humanity.

When I returned to the house, I took a hot shower and enjoyed a lovely dinner of soup, fresh bread, and a green salad with my hosts and their young friend, Amanda. We laughed and talked. After dinner, we all snuggled up on the big white couch and watched *Thelma and Louise* choose to live and die, again.

Water, Water Everywhere

When God decides to baptize you, it's not just a few hours in a church on a Sunday afternoon. For me, it was a seasonal production; that autumn I began to see the element of water at every turn.   I was completely captivated by it. Sitting by rivers, streams, oceans, and puddles, I found myself immersed in the tension at the surface of water everywhere. I began to imagine the dark place under the water as the earthly world and the air above the water as a spirit world. Where those two worlds met was the surface—a third world of reflection. The unique tension at the surface of water was formed by both worlds and simultaneously transcended both worlds. The supposedly flat surface of water became a new doorway as I imagined a whole different reality being born, opening up like a tear in the fabric of space. Suddenly water was referenced in every written passage my eyes gazed on. I read articles, books, and poems about water. Movies contained watery metaphors, and the multifaceted liquid seemed to be the subject of all visual arts. I waded in brooks and sat by rivers. I found lessons in every stream.

The Charles River ran through two consecutive weekends of Zero Balancing classes. In late October, Dr. Smith was teaching an advanced class, the Alchemy of Touch, at St. Stephen's Priory in Dover, Massachusetts. The priory was less than five miles from my childhood home—only a mile by the river. As a youngster, I rode my bicycle over the undulating back roads between my home and the priory. My father often put his canoe in the Charles River at Route 27 and the stretch of river from there to the priory was the usual Sunday afternoon paddle. In high school, my friends and I drove along the railroad tracks, parked the car, crept across the thirty-foot high trestle that spanned the river, and hiked up to the granite outcropping called Rocky Ledges to drink beer and flirt with each other. The serpent of my life was eating its own tail. My past came full circle with my present in the current of that meandering river, as ZB and my esteemed teacher came to my childhood stomping ground.

Each day at lunchtime during the class, I shuffled my way through six fluffy inches of fallen leaves down the path to the river. There is something a little sassy about walking through fallen leaves. There is no doing it silently so I figured I might as well revel in the cacophony of my unashamed human presence and the sweet, dry aroma of autumnal decay. I kicked the leaves up and threw them overhead as I walked. When I got to the river, I found it was still the river of my childhood—both the same and different. The inevitability of the flow was both comforting and fascinating. I watched as leaves of the holy oaks were released, swirled gracefully down to the water's surface, and were swept away in the current to new adventures. Time was both standing still and moving on. Once again, a new dimension popped open, plumper than the one from which I had emerged. Images were more defined, colors were brighter, and the world was more alive. I felt as if the water had the potential to teach me all that there was to know. I absorbed the truth of the world through all my sensory channels: everything is as it should be.

The following weekend, I attended another ZB class in *Water*town, Massachusetts, of all places. Having become a certified Zero Balancing practitioner, I was invited by my teacher, Jim, to assist in teaching the basic program. The class was held in a large brick building perched on the side of the Charles River. Behind the building, there was a small park and walking path that followed along the river. I brought my lunch each day and sat on a park bench enjoying the roar of the water spilling over the herring run, watching cormorants preen and ducks...well...duck. The calendar had shed its vibrant orange October leaf, and the raw gray edge of November was exposed. The water seeped deeper into my bones.

Simultaneously observing the natural world with my senses and experiencing myself unified with it, I became a child perceiving the world anew. *Ah, this is the gift of Eden*, I thought. *When duality and unity are held simultaneously, a portal to innocence is opened.* A diagram surfaced from that portal:

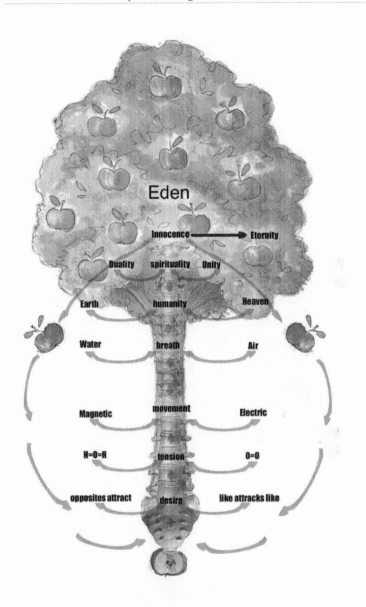

I didn't know exactly what it meant, but the feeling that everything had its place was undeniable. It occurred to me that this strange new diagram is shaped like the human brain. Is there a reason our brains are shaped like this? Is there a seed of our innocence programmed into our physiological development, creating the potential for the return to Eden? Is life a virtual joyride around our cerebral hemispheres? Have we developed our brains by the very process of splitting from Eden and trying to get back to One?

My experience from this birth is *Yes*—yes to all questions and all possibilities. Yes. Yes. Yes. I am not limited to what is scientifically proven. I am evolving through the need to have someone verify who I am, how I'm made, and whether my experience is correct or not. Yes. It is. If I suffer, there is a way to peace: back to Eden, through the eyes of a child, the eyes of innocence.

By the time I took my leave of the Charles River, it had sucked me in completely, swallowed my flesh, and spit out the bones:

Eden

I breathe
at the river's edge.
I move
in the reflection
and dance
in the distance in
between.

All beauty surrounds
me now.

> I rise
> to the innocent
> Eden.
> Eternity beats
> my heart
> and gives birth to me,
> my child.

Checking in with Jim after the Watertown class, I shared my sudden obsession and fascination with water. He told me that in Chinese medicine the water element is the deepest element, the element related to winter, when the sap goes deep inside. It is related to the essence that we receive from our parents when we are conceived, to the bones, to our deepest spirits, to wisdom, and to letting our lives be in harmony with the unfolding of our true nature.

Very cool! I am being reborn from the ashes of my own bones and the teacher, the element of water, reaches out to me and pulls me in to winter, showing me my deepest essence is innocence. I don't even have to know anything about Chinese medicine. Everything I need to know is programmed in to the very world in which I exist and the sensory apparatus that is my body.

Touching Water

Sometimes in autumn, the foliage is at its most colorful but the experience is dampened by rainy, raw, or blustery weather. At other times there may be a stretch of days when the foliage is at its peak, and the sky is clear and sunny with just enough of a breeze to kiss cheeks and make them blush. The sight of translucent reds, yellows, and oranges backlit against a brilliant blue sky sends endorphins squirting into the bloodstream. On those days it's hard for me to do anything but look with wonder at the world and inhale endlessly in to the sublime longing at the bottom of my heart. It was on one of these stunning fall days that I set off on a solitary walk through the village of Wilmington, up the long slope of Castle Hill to Lake Whitingham. When I arrived, I found the lake immersed in the still, silent awe of her role as the lap of profound beauty, holding a mirror to the flaming shore. We all (the trees, the lake, and I) beheld the splendor doubled in her crystal clear reflection.

It was so serene I could hear the trees whisper to each other. They were showing off for me. "Here comes the girl," they whispered, as they admired themselves in the mirror. "Everybody sparkle! Stand up tall. Brighten. She sees our beauty. Come on. Shine! Give it your all!"

Tears gathered at the edge of my lower eyelid. *They are trying for me! They are giving to me. They see me.* Now, while it is apparently not the nature of most trees to sprout faces and start talking like the ones in *The Wizard of OZ*, although sometimes I still look for that kind of thing, trees do talk in a different way. Trees talk within themselves. I have found that if I am quiet and if my mind is free, their words will come and climb inside me, and I will know. When I ask for the medicine of plants and animals, it finds me. That's how Eden found me.

I wanted to touch the beauty with my hands. *Which is more real—the world reflected on the surface or the world above the surface?* Crouching down, I peered into the water. The bottom of the lake, usually visible through six to eight feet of clear water, was hidden behind a new world of unquenchable color. Slowly, I stretched my open palms toward the mirrored surface. The simple act of touching water became a spontaneously sacred ritual. I watched myself moving in slow motion despite my usual avoidance of ceremonial dramatics. My hands instinctively knew how to approach the house of God: slowly, carefully, and with heightened awareness. The lake, like a lover, was showing me how to touch her. *I want to feel who she is. I am using my ZB touch. All of my awareness is in my fingers and on the intention of interface.* The closer my hands came to the water, the slower they moved as if anticipating the meeting. What would it feel like to arrive at the interface of air and water, of object and reflection? What would it feel like to arrive at the interface of heaven and earth? When there was less than an eighth of an inch between the water and me, it strained to jump up and meet me. Someplace between what was the surface and what was me, we met in an explosion of sensation that was electric, fluid, sharp, clear, giving, and vibrant. All the sensory receptors in my palms began to dance like the keys on a player piano. The cold fire of vitality poured into my hands, up through my arms, and into all of me. It was not the old wet and cold sensation of water. The thin document of conditioned knowing gave way to lush innocent perception. It was so much more than I had previously known. It was true beauty and consummate bliss. *This is what it feels like to be alive. This is what it feels like to be awake.*

The Invitation

Sometimes we are just standing too close to ourselves. In the middle of my life, I found I was beside myself while watching myself trying to become something I already was. I kept looking past myself to find the divine while she was relaxing in the soft folds of my flesh waiting to be invited into my awareness.

Throughout most spiritual traditions there is the practice and promise of prayer: ask and you shall receive. Yet many people feel their prayers go unanswered. Prayer is the invitation to communication with our higher power and communication is a two way street. Perhaps all prayers would be answered if we allowed them to be, if we truly let them be. In Genesis, the first book of the Bible, God invites the world into being: "and the Spirit of God was moving over the surface of the waters. And God said, 'Let there be light'; and there was light."[3]

Paul McCartney and John Lennon wrote in the classic Beatles song:

"And when the broken hearted people living in the world agree,
there will be an answer, Let it Be.
And when the night is cloudy there is still a light that shines on me,
there will be an answer, Let it Be."[4]

Allow, open, and invite. In his teachings of the Sufi's mystical journey, Llewellyn Vaughan-Lee writes that when we walk toward God, God comes running to us. And when a human being opens her heart, dedicates her life to the service of God, and is prepared to sacrifice her ego to the truth of love, creation conspires to help her in every way. She will meet with the assistance of many hands—seen and unseen.[5]

In the Native American path, opening to the *energy* of the animals, plants, and ancestors, in addition to acknowledging their structural presence, invites the offering of their medicine. They will council, guide, and teach if asked.

If I invite spirit in to my life and let it live in me and let it be me, then there is grace.
Emmylou Harris sings:

"And when Mother Mary finally comes to call
She could pass right through your heart
And leave no trace at all
While you were reaching for
The sacred and the divine
She was standing right beside you
All the time".[6]

So, here within the acute context of family, we invited Eden to live among us even as we lived within her. What were we inviting? A permanent wound? No. The memory of a potential child, a possible sibling? Not so much. The spirit of a being that had come to answer my prayers? More likely.

Prayers are answered. It is just that so often the answer comes in an unrecognizable form. I asked for more connection to the divine. I let myself wonder what it would be like to be consciously pregnant. And here, through loss, grief, and disappointment is a connection to the other world. I thought I wanted to be connected to a more divine place through the hand of God in my belly. But the God in my belly was showing me that it was just a delusion that I was ever disconnected. With the acceptance of the separation of this baby and me, I gained the awareness that the divine and I would never be and have never been separate.

Eden is the garden of innocence; it's the place of perfection that is left behind and lost to humans who strive for knowledge as an accumulation of facts. Eden is the forest that humans lose sight of when they stand too close to their perception that we are individual trees competing for sunlight. Eden was not born into an earthly body. He is not male or female. She would not be on earth or in heaven. He resides in Eden, which is the place before knowledge brought duality. She teaches us that all exists in unity. Eden is a baby. Eden is a spirit. Eden is a child and a parent. He was birthed by me and she birthed me. Eden becomes so much more as I continue to learn from a place of innocence and trust: trust that all is as it should be and that our prayers are answered. The world offers up a different face when we trust that the answer we receive is what is best for us, and when we practice real, live, living trust in God.

Police

Sometimes an alternate reality seeps through the veil between worlds and cuts you off.   It's kind of a crash between two worlds.   You know these times because they are so bizarre or surreal that they literally come out of left field.

It was around Halloween, All Hallows Eve in the pagan tradition, when the spirit world is closest to the physical world, and we can more easily see through the mists that separate us.   Three months had passed since the birth and death of Eden.   Dale was back on the road, and Justin was in school.   Beau and I had been out of town getting an unusually early start on Christmas shopping.   Returning home, I pulled into the driveway to see an unfamiliar car sitting there.   I did not have office hours that day but thought perhaps it was a patient waiting to pick up vitamins, pay a bill, or make an appointment.

I extricated Beau from his car seat and unloaded the bags from the back of the car, figuring whoever it was would make his or her purpose known as I approached. After dropping the bags in the foyer and settling a sleepy Beau on the couch for a nap, I returned to the front porch to greet the visitors.   A local police officer and another man were walking up the front walk.

"Hello, Mrs. Doucette, I'm Sergeant Jack Thomson from the Wilmington Police Department and this is Detective Wilson from the Vermont State Police.   We'd like to ask you some questions."

"Okay," I said lightly, "Why don't you go in through my office door and wait for me there. I am going to check on my son, and I'll be right over."

Interesting. Maybe they are investigating some happening in town or something to do with one of my patients? Well, whatever it is, I don't know anything juicy, so I am sure it will be short and simple.

I entered the office still rustling like the crisp brown maple leaves that whirled and skipped as I drove up the driveway moments earlier. Jack was sitting in a straight back chair looking slightly sheepish; the detective was perched on the window seat looking smug.

"Sorry to keep you waiting. I just got home from Christmas shopping. How can I help you?" I blurted cheerfully, trying to settle into being present with them.

They both smiled politely, well actually, patronizingly. Detective Wilson began. "Mrs. Doucette…"

I don't like being called Mrs. Doucette. I am commonly referred to as either Michele or Dr. Doucette. Being called Mrs. Doucette feels like having my name mispronounced; it just doesn't catch my attention or make a direct connection to who I am.

He continued, "Is it true that you had a miscarriage earlier this year?"

Boom. He came crashing into my lane. Now he had my attention. The atmosphere in the room became heavy and I retreated somewhere into the back of my ribcage.

"Yes," was the obvious answer and I offered it tentatively.

"And how far along were you…."

I veered over and crashed back into him. "Okay..so..what's this all about?" I said sharply. "Let's get to the point right now because you're freaking me out."

The contents of my vehicle, the molecules of my emotions, were bouncing off of each other like Ping-Pong balls in a lottery machine.

"It is my duty to investigate unreported deaths, and we are trying to determine…."

"You have no idea what you're doing!" I warned him.

All the Ping-Pong balls were vying for the escape hatch, and I didn't know which one would spring first.

"Well, we'd just like to know…," he tried to continue evenly.

"How dare you!" I cried. "You have no idea what you are doing!" The first winning lottery number tonight is: RAGE. "Where did this come from? This is a very personal, very feminine matter! You have no idea," I repeated.

"I know this is a sensitive matter…"

My defenses softened a little as I realized that he actually *didn't* know that he was trampling on holy ground. He was coming from another world.

"You don't know me," I said, more to myself than to him. Equanimity and understanding were settling in. Forgiveness was already making her sweet appearance. "You don't know me," I whispered, tears spilling onto my cheeks. I turned to Jack feeling naked and beaten. "What? How did this come down?"

He spoke for the first time. "It came to my attention that there was a miscarriage and that you buried the child on your property. I was unsure of how to proceed, so I contacted the State Police."

I could imagine some bosomy, busybody, insipid soccer mom or shopkeeper whipping up a story. Any news is good news in a small town. "Christ. Who told you that? Whose business is it?"

"I really can't say...I..."

"Nevermind. It doesn't matter. Jesus Christ, Jack."

I turned back to the detective. "What do you want to know?" I asked with resignation. The wave of rage had passed for the moment, but my teeth were still chattering.

"How far along was the pregnancy when you miscarried?"

"Four months," I said quietly.

"Were you under medical care?"

What does this man know about pregnancy? Probably nothing. I felt sickened by the presence of two men questioning if how I dealt with my pregnancy was appropriate. I was offended as a physician and as woman. *How dare they sit here and question me from some illusory position of power? The least they could have done was to send a woman.*

"I had just been to my midwife for the first visit the week before. There was no heartbeat."

His face hardened. "Why didn't you go to the hospital?"

Rage, round two. "Why?! To have my dead baby sucked out of me by some machine and thrown into a container labeled medical waste? Why would anyone want to do *that*?"

A wave of sorrow rose in my heart. *That's not the way to honor life.* Then, the gentle momentum of that one sorrowful wave sucked all the sediment off the ocean floor. Eons of feminine sadness, loss, loneliness, and frustration, compressed by the weight of misunderstanding, oppression, denigration, and violation, exploded through the aqueduct of my usual reserve. Tears like hot lava streamed down my face.

"This is sacred ground," I warned again. The rage was ancient and archetypical, the power of the divine female rising to full height. I was Kali, the goddess of creation and destruction. And the wave passed.

"I'm sorry. You just don't know," I said into the air.

Rage and forgiveness were dancing a tango in my heart. Maybe someplace between the two these men could hear the truth and learn.

Integrity. Hold integrity. They don't know. For all this guy knows I could be some drug addict mother flushing my kids down the toilet. Or maybe I was a member of a secret baby-killing cult. I'll give him some credit, though. State policemen typically do not do well when repeatedly told they don't know what they're doing. Now, there is no excuse for the local policeman letting it go this far. We've lived and worked in this small community for years. Our children go to the same school. Has he no intuition? No ability to judge character? Was the gossip just too much to resist? Even if it was his duty, couldn't he have called with a caring word and told me the situation left some questions in his lap? No excuse. Police protocol or not, bad move, Jack.

After a short silence the detective spoke again, "I'd like to talk to your doctor. We need to determine if there was actually a birth because if there was, we would have to document a death."

"And just what *is* the criterion here?" I challenged quickly. "At what point is a fetus born and at what point is the product of a miscarriage just medical waste?"

I could sense his position of authority weaken, and I thought I could hear his inner voice reiterating a motto of detective training. *Maintain authority at all times when questioning suspects.*

"I don't know if there is an established criterion," he said thoughtfully. "It may be the viability of the life of the child outside of the mother."

Good answer. I'll give him that. Good answer.

I looked him in the eye steadily, raised my hand up beside my face, and spread my thumb and index finger three inches apart. "It was this big. It wasn't viable," I said authoritatively, with just a twist of bitterness. "But, sure, go ask my doctor. Why should you believe me? Right? Sorry. Whatever!"

You either know the truth right now, or you wouldn't know the truth if it bit you in the ass.

****

Mary phoned me from her office a few hours later.

"Hello?"

"Hi, Michele, it's Mary," she said gently.   There was one of those five-second pauses that seem so vast. "Are you okay?"

"Yeah, I'm all right."

"Jesus."

"I know."

Round Two

When one journey ends another begins. Life is an unending spiral. I thought the physical part of the pregnancy was over with the burial of Eden, but the nine-month cycle of gestation continued. On January 4th, my original due date, I was working in my office. I had evaluated my patient in the seated position and asked him to lay face down on the adjusting table. After he settled himself on the table, I began to evaluate his lower back. Suddenly, I felt my life force drain downward and pour out of me with one sudden flush. It was as if my water broke. My legs wobbled, and my head swirled. I could not finish the appointment. Excusing myself, I stumbled out of the room, and while blindly passing by Denise, asked her to deal with the patient.

When labor begins there is no going back, and with this one, there was not even any break between contractions. I contracted into severe illness for five days. I have never been so sick. I was weak, extremely nauseous, and freezing cold. My head was so painful that it was easy to imagine giving up on this life just to escape the torment. I was so cold I had to wear a winter hat to bed and have the down comforter pulled completely over me just to get the minimal amount of sleep that I managed. I rocked back and forth to distract myself. I said, "I'm so sick" endlessly. It was a sickness mantra chanted not so much for self pity as for survival.   Repeating the words seemed to be a mechanism to remember that this was just a state of illness, this was not me. Acknowledging the suffering allowed me to hang on to the healthy essence that was beneath it. It allowed me to be both whole and broken. It was my breath work for a labor I thought had long past.

I awoke to the third sunrise, and the pain and nausea still had not subsided. I sent Dale out for some over-the-counter medication. I hadn't taken anything besides herbs and homeopathic remedies for more than fifteen years. I guess this was the point in a normal hospital birth where I might have accepted an epidural. I was not trying to be heroic by avoiding drugs. It was my belief that pharmaceutical drugs were toxic, and it was my experience that my body knew how to heal anything that needed healing. Now I was so tired of the pain and so weak that I needed relief to stay connected to that healthy me underneath. Dale brought home some antihistamine that seemed to dull the pain so I could get more sleep. I stayed in bed for two more days with my son's winter hat on.

I had no baby, but just to be sure I was still paying attention, I was given the pain of labor again. There was something a *lot* bigger than my own personal drama unfolding here.

Falling to pieces

Sometimes in the wholeness of life, I fall to pieces.
Several months after my due-date flu, my hair began to
fall out. Considering the cycle of the pregnancy, I was
three months postpartum. Okay, about three months
after having a baby, my hair *would* be falling out. But it
was more hair loss than I remembered from my previous
two births. I was also experiencing headaches, fatigue,
loss of appetite, and a ghostly thin feeling. I was
slipping away—living on air and adrenaline, dehydrated,
and disappearing into the ether. I tried to surrender into
the postpartum story, but it wasn't the right story, or,
more likely, it wasn't the whole story.

Toward the end of March, I traveled to Connecticut
to assist Jim teach another Zero Balancing class. I was
attentive to my health but not committed to the idea that
it was anything more than a passing phase. I was
watching my situation unfold. Interestingly, during that
particular course, I had decided to work on improving
my eyesight. Anytime I work with ZB, whether
receiving a session or teaching, I work strongly with
intention. Previously I had read a little about natural
vision improvement. I wanted to investigate whether or
not I could improve my eyesight by removing my lenses
and glasses, and focusing my attention on what was
there to see and by softening my vision and being more
receptive. I was also aware that perhaps there was
something I didn't want to see and so had narrowed my
vision subconsciously. The hair loss issue hadn't quite

solidified into something around which I could build an intention for this class. So, the eyes would have it. Surprisingly, even though I had learned to expect such synchronicities in the world of ZB, there were a few other students in this large class who were also exploring their eyesight.

Whenever there is attention from multiple sources coming together, there is a greater possibility for change. In a classroom situation, there is a certain amount of group energy or chi cultivated by the instructors and students as they share and expand their knowledge and experience of a particular subject. When all of that energy is directed to a particular theory or practice, there is the possibility for the learning to go deeper and be more powerful. Imagine feeling all the love (a type of energy) from the people closest to your heart, coming to you from wherever those people are at the moment, despite any other activities that they may be engaged in. It is possible to feel their love. Now, imagine you bring them all together to be in the very same room with you. Tell them your intention is to be able to feel all the love you share with them. Maybe one is mother love, one is a friend, a lover, or a teacher. Maybe someone thinks the whole thing is a lousy idea and isn't really able to concentrate his or her energy in this way. Still, the field is amplified for your intention.

This particular class was pretty intense. Largely composed of physical therapists from an expansive alternative medicine facility, the group was extremely knowledgeable and detail oriented. The classroom was charged equally with the passion and the pride this group had for their particular kind of work. Sometimes when the mind is accustomed to driving, it is challenging to drop down to what's happening underneath the awareness of knowledge— what the brazilian novelist, Paulo Coelho, calls "the soul of the world."[7]

In the soul of the world is where Zero Balancing shines. It is where ZB moves, deep in the marrow, the juicy depths of the bone, underneath the conscious mind, underneath the emotions and conditioning, and underneath the ego. I felt the group dynamic in this class was such that we were just grazing the periosteum, the soft outer layer of bone, a tissue more involved with defining the mind's knowledge of the soul than experiencing the soul directly. ZB offers us the opportunity to dig our eyeteeth into the bone.

I became aware of resistance to the marrow when I offered help to one student who quickly put his hand up in front of my face as if to say *stop*. "This is the way I do it," he said. A familiar feeling of fragility arose. It might have been a clue that something was cooking in my bones.

Later that evening, my fellow assistant Verilee, Jim, and I met at our hotel to trade ZB sessions. It would be a fun way to spend the evening; we'd do some ZB and afterward go out to dinner. When it was my turn on the table, I reiterated my frame; I wanted to be able to soften my focus, widen my vision, and see whatever I had not been able to see. As I lay down, the image of the student's hand raised to refuse my help re-appeared, and the fragile feeling returned. It seemed to be bringing to my awareness so much more than a no thanks. I was hearing, "Don't touch me. I don't want to listen to you. I don't want you."

Not long after settling on to the table, anticipating the deep satisfaction of the ZB touch, I became agitated by the tension building around my eyes and brow. I mentioned it to Jim, and he moved to the head of the table and put his hands on my head. I was blindsided by a wave of sadness that seemed to be pouring out of my skin as if I were sweating tears. Simultaneously, there was a flash of an image. I could feel my closed eyelids fluttering, which is a sign that I was entering an altered state of consciousness. Jim asked what was going on. I told him that I was feeling profound sadness. Knowing that the fleeting image was probably important, I willed myself to drop down deeper into the feeling of sadness to retrieve the information within.

Suddenly, I was an infant lying in one of those raised hospital carts they put newborns in. It was hard and foreign. I was isolated. I was swaddled tightly in a blanket. Large, indifferent pieces of metal machinery stood watch from various outposts on the perimeter of the room. The people were distant and distracted. I sensed the proximity of my mother's body, but she was not aware of me. We were unplugged from each other. All of my awareness was behind my eyes. I couldn't move my body. *Would someone please look into my eyes? I need connection. I need to feel that I have arrived somewhere. There is no landing for me. I need to see the God in some other eyes. I need reflection. I'm alone.* There was only busyness and business.

I narrated my experience to Jim in some form, and he held the helm quietly for a few moments. "Is there anything else?"

I searched my awareness, always the good student, wanting to get as much from my session as possible. *Anger? No, move away from anger. Anger? No, I shouldn't be angry at her. She's my mother, and she didn't know. That's just how they did it then—with general anesthesia. I love my mom! Anger? Okay, if it knocks three times, listen. Okay, Anger.*

"A little anger, I guess," I said meekly. *Suppress anger.*

"Can you tell me more about that?" Jim asked evenly.

There was a pause in which I had to consider the truth. *Mother anger— it's so cliché. Oh well, let's see what it's all about.*

"I feel angry at my mother that she wasn't there." Ugh.

"Is there anything you would like to do with that anger?"

I paused to consider the truth. "No. It was like archetypical anger or something. It's like watching a passing realization. I just didn't know that it was ever in me."

"Yeah."

While I was watching the anger being gently washed from my interior with the tide, I was suddenly lifted and tossed over by a big wave of laughter—the doubling-over kind of uncontrollable, tear-inducing belly laughter. I guess it was infectious laugher because

I could hear Jim and Verilee getting caught up in the wave with giggles. A miniature Joni Mitchell sang inside my head, "laughing and crying, you know it's the same release."[8] After a minute or two the wave passed.

In his compassionate tone, with hint of a smile still lingering in his voice, Jim asked, "What's happening?"

"I don't know. It's just so funny." Another wave of deep laughter rolled in.

"*What* is so funny?" he said softly.

"I don't know. The laughter is just happening. I mean it's kind of funny that we were just going to do a little ZB and have some dinner, and I get on the table and casually have this little rebirth experience." More laughter. "Where the hell did *that* come from?"
I was laughing with the release and with my continued amazement at the power of ZB.

"Well, where *did* it come from?"

I quieted. My eyeballs were moving quickly from side to side behind closed lids. I was searching the invisible files of my subconscious for the answer. "I guess I needed to see what happened at my birth." I continued searching files. "And probably from my miscarriage."

"Yeah."

Fields of Life and Death

After the ZB rebirth session, Jim excused himself from our dinner plans. Maybe he was tired after a long day as teacher and midwife. Maybe he knew it was important for me to have time to integrate. Maybe I was in shock. I remember the look on my babies' faces when they were born. It was a sleepy taking-it-all-for-granted type of surprise. If they could have verbalized it, it may have sounded something like "everything is as it should be, as it always is, and always will be, and holy cow, where the heck am I now?" I think I must have looked something like that.

Still feeling numb from the anesthesia of birth, I made my way down the corridor to my hotel room. My hand reached out to insert the key card, and the door clicked open. I sat on the end of a bed draped in buoyant, floral synthetic. The walls were dark green with ambiguous artwork hanging in predictable places. A stiff chair sat by a small desk waiting for the phone to ring. This place gave me no visual, olfactory, auditory, or tactile sense of where I was. My mind knew that I was in a hotel room somewhere in Connecticut, but my body was suspended in nothingness. Maybe it was all divinely planned; this was the perfect neutral environment to begin to understand what this session, this rebirth, was all about. There had been no one there to reach out to me with recognition of spirit when I was born. This room reflected that lack of presence and vitality. It was void. I was void. I was alone. I wasn't going to wait for the chair to receive her call. She might as well realize that she was alone, too. I butted in and called Dale.

"Hello?" he answered.

"Hi, sweetie. How's it going?"

"Well, actually, I've had a very bizarre day," he said tentatively, maybe a bit defensively.

"What's going on?"

"Ah…well… everything started off normally. I made the kids breakfast and got them off to school. Everything was good. It was a nice day. I started to clean up the house. I was sweeping the kitchen floor when I got this feeling that I was going to die."

Diagnostic mode kicked in. "What do you mean by going to die? Like having chest pain or weakness? What did you feel?"

"I don't know. I just had this overwhelming sense that I was going to die. I had to stop sweeping and go outside. I sat out back on the porch swing for a while and just told myself to breathe. After a while, I started to feel a little better and went back to cleaning the house, but the feeling came on again just as strong." He hesitated. "I thought you put a hex on me, and I was going to die. I know it's weird, but that's just what I was thinking. I went back outside and had to just sit there for a while. It happened a few more times after that."

"A *hex* on you? Why would I put a hex on you? Why would you think that? I don't even *do* hexes!"

"I know. I don't know. It was really weird."

We were both silent for a bit.

"And how are you now?"

"Okay...I mean I feel pretty normal, but a little shaken up, I guess."

"Do you know that I love you? And I would never put a hex on you even if I did hexes?" I said in my cutest you-love-me-don't-you kind of voice that makes Dale smile.

"Yeah, I guess," he answered dryly.

"WHAT?"

"Yeah, I *know*. It's just been a weird day."

"Why do you think that happened?" I asked.

"I have no idea."

"I do. Can I tell you what just happened to *me*?"

"Sure."

I narrated my ZB session to Dale as he listened quietly. "So, it seems," I said, "that I was being reborn, and you were dying. I doubt that's a coincidence. I mean, you're my other half. If some awareness deep within one of us is shifting, it makes sense that something would have to happen to the other person. You know, that equal and opposite reaction thing?"

"Hmmm..."

"What do you think about that?"

"I don't know what to think. Interesting idea, I guess. I don't really know what it all means," he said slowly. "But, if you're going to do something like that again, can you give me a little more warning next time?"

****

My latest ZB session helped to open an opportunity, a

space within myself to reprogram beliefs that no longer served me. The session took me, as ZB often does, underneath my daily awareness and into my bones, my cement, and my foundation. There I found separation from God at birth, separation from my mother, separation from the matrix of life as I had previously known it. Going into the bone, I mined the bitter mineral of separation imprinted in my dark underground. I stepped into the black hole of isolation and fell into the vibration of separation. Two hundred miles north and hours earlier, my husband felt the life force pull away from him. He felt his impending death was related to me. His mind began to formulate ways in which I could influence his death from afar. His mind was inaccurate, his feelings were spot on.

Michael Faraday described field theory in the late nineteenth century. It is no great news to physicists around the world that electromagnetic fields exist and interact. It is common scientific knowledge that events occurring in one part of a field affect other parts of that field in nonlocal and nonlinear ways. Human beings emit electromagnetic fields and are part of fields larger than themselves. An individual does not have to understand field theory to experience its truth; most people have encountered events that are remarkably and uncannily connected. These matters of coincidence should not be dismissed as trivial anomalies. Something right happens when we look for the connection.

Resonant DNA

Sitting on the sidelines at a third grade basketball game one day, I realized my weekly transformation into loud sports mom was more than simple zeal for my son's athletic development. Why is it so hard to sit quietly and politely like some of the other moms, and watch eight-year-old children cavort up and down the basketball court with their arms and legs flailing and wobbling on the edge of self-control? How is it that a mild-mannered nature enthusiast finds herself folded over the boards in a hockey rink barking "suggestions" at her son who knows ten times as much about ice hockey as she does? What is it that makes me want to jump through the skin of my progeny as they exert themselves but watching strangers play leaves me unaffected (except, of course, when the New England Patriots win the Superbowl)?

Resonant DNA. It must be. It's the only explanation for the utter transformation between the first whistle and the final buzzer. There must be something that resonates between my sons and me at such times. I think it is the way we are encoded. Perhaps our DNA is a not only the structural blueprint for the expression our physical characteristics, but also the energetic, vibrational score of our own personal symphony. The nucleotides that line themselves up along the double helixes of our DNA may encode the expression of eye color, but the spaces between the genes may offer the rhythm, the movement, and desires of those eyes:

green-eyed female, likes to dance, would rather skip than run, and cannot drive fifty-five.

For my part, I seem to be wired for short bursts of fluid activity punctuated by connection, acknowledgement, and containment. The same genes that specifically encoded long, lean muscles and broad shoulders may also be causative in their orientation to what feels good to that structure. Whatever energy, vibration, rhythm is in phase with that structure is what feels good to me. I imagine the gene sequence in my cells. Maybe it looks something like this:

GCATGGCATGGCAAAAATGGGAAA

The letters signify the sequence of the specific bases that are attached to the double helix. Maybe the sequence of CAT determines that I will have red hair. Maybe it is junk DNA, a term for sequences of bases that do not encode any particular physical characteristic. But maybe the junk functions in the encoding of our energy, our movement, our rhythms, and the expression of our vitality. The placement and resulting cadence of the CAT sequence could be responsible for the fact that I delight in the rhythm of two short "notes" followed by a longer or more intense note.

I long for the *stroke, kick, KICK* of the Butterfly stroke in swimming, the *bump, set, SPIKE* of a competitive volleyball match, the *chicka, chicka, BOOM* of a good rock beat. Perhaps the junk DNA is holding the space—a place from which to hear ourselves. I used to jog regularly because I liked the strength I developed from it. I tolerate it much less as time passes because it is so ultimately boring to me. Step after step without a pause or playful curve is just too predictable. I find myself stopping to look more closely at a beautiful plant, to put my hands in the cool stream, or to listen to animal voices and receive their medicine. I need the pause to listen, to reflect, and to learn. I imagine if one's gene sequence is more regular or repetitive, it may feel great to run marathons, to listen to feet, and breaths continue in regular cadence.

Playing the music of their resonant DNA, my children awaken my music. They create vibration and movement within me. I want to pass, run, and jump; I want to skate, shoot, and score. But I am sitting on the sidelines trying to be a spectator and contain the game being played deep within my cells. So, I cheer, whoop, and holler. It is, truly, the least I can do.

Eyes

When Eden was born, the light of his soul was not behind those tiny eyes. Her eyes were closed in peaceful slumber—the peace that exists beneath the drama of human life. The peace that feels like all is well, that all is love. Still, I yearn to look into those eyes and recognize the awareness of heaven touching earth. This presence was in the eyes of my sons when they were born: peaceful, steady, freshly awakened, though I don't know that I was present enough then to bring full awareness to what I was seeing.

With Justin, I was twenty-eight and just beginning my internship in chiropractic school. He conveniently dropped into the world in the pause between the end of classes and the beginning of final exams. He was welcomed to life and held in the compassionate hands of the Los Angeles College of Chiropractic class of December 1989. Having learned to crawl in the halls of the school clinic, Justin has an easy social grace and a profound appreciation for office supplies. We have been a faithful companions and loyal friends from the beginning.

When Beau was born, I was thirty-three and at the height of my personal expression, building a practice, competing in triathlons, backpacking in the wilderness with him four months in my belly. Beau embodies that enthusiasm, that adventurous spirit, and that love of the physical. He is intensely sensitive, competitive, and ready to try anything.

I was thirty-nine with Eden. Astrologically, this is in the midst of Uranus opposition, at the intersection of the first and second halves of my life, where the infinity symbol of my life meets itself. It was the time of my own rebirth. I was ready to see, to re-experience and to re-pattern. And isn't that just what she offered? If I had seen the spark of light in his eyes, it would still have been in *his* eyes. It would still have been separate from my own experience. *I* was to be Eden's eyes. The point was not merely to look on this divine state of being but to be it. It was not to look on God within another being but to be in union with God within my own flesh.

I guess it was in fourth grade, when my eyesight became strained, and my perspective was lost on another level. I was required to recite the answers to math facts on sight. I was expected to read color-coded booklets in far less time than I actually could and answer questions about the content. It was horrifying trying to read under pressure. My eyes began to sabotage me; the faster I tried to read, the more fixed and halting they became. By the fourth grade, I had learned there was a world of fixed and predetermined knowledge external to me. It had nothing to do with the soft, fluid soup of feelings I carried around inside my warm little body. I learned that if I was good enough and smart enough, if I worked hard enough, someday I would understand or even master that world. As my focus shifted toward external achievement, my vision blurred and doubled. Eyeglass lenses became a permanent filter between the incongruities of the outer world and the world behind my eyes.

Are lenses protective eye-wear that help me to bring focus back to this illusion of the world I create? Do sharply defined borders keep us believing in our separation from the rest of life? Who is to say it is more correct that there is only a singular dotted line riding down the center of the road than the two I see without lenses?   If everyone who wore eyeglasses stopped wearing them, would they evolve their sight perception and other perceptive faculties so that the world we agree on would be more variable, more multidimensional? Or would we all just crash into each other? It's hard to know. What I do know is that I trust this ZB experience. I asked what I was not seeing and the answer was given. It was Eden, the blurred edge between heaven and earth.

Purgatory

The daily tangle on my hairbrush was growing bigger.
Long spiraled strands would just fall in my lap now and
then. Every time I swept my hair back off my face, I
would have to shake individual curls off of my hand.
The daily headaches and heavy fatigue continued. It
was all too clear to me that my health was suffering. I
decided I needed to be responsible for my health. I
define *responsible* as the ability to respond. I had to look
the situation in the face to know how to respond. I
needed information. I consulted my trusted naturopath,
Mary, and we embarked on a course of investigation.
After taking a thorough history of my situation, Mary
drew blood for a complete blood count (CBC), arthritis
panel, thyroid tests, and heavy-metal toxicity analysis.
This would give us a place to start.

The first round of tests revealed a normal blood
count, normal thyroid levels, rheumatoid factor:
negative, sedimentation rate: elevated, and a positive
ANA (antinuclear antibody) titer. An elevated
sedimentation rate is a general indication of an active
inflammatory process. A positive ANA is a somewhat
more specific test indicating the body is making
antibodies to its own self. This was not particularly
good news; an autoimmune condition was what I feared.
My mother has an autoimmune condition known as
discoid lupus. She has had an immune reaction to her
own skin. Fortunately, it is isolated to her skin, and she
has never developed systemic lupus, which can destroy

organs and muscles. My mother had lost much of her hair at about my age. With all of my training over the years, I was repeatedly exposed to the knowledge that autoimmune diseases are often hereditary, but I never took it in. I never heard that *I* was susceptible to an autoimmune disease because I was never approaching forty years of age— the time in life when the lacquered finish of invincibility begins to peel and flake.

Maybe I had lupus. Maybe I would lose all my hair and would have to wear a synthetic wig on my head. (I don't even wear synthetic fabric in my clothing!) Would it block the universal life flow of energy coming into the crown of my head? I could shave my head and be bald, wear dangly earrings, and be *tres chic*. I thought of all the brave women undergoing chemotherapy who had lost their hair. I cried at the thought of losing my femininity with my hair. My mind went through all the options and scenarios at record speed. Did I have systemic lupus? Was it possible that my heart was being eaten up or that my kidneys were shutting down? Would I have to tell my boys that their mama was dying?

Was it another cycle of death and rebirth, or a final death? If we keep moving, do we ever really experience death as an end? Does life keep reinventing itself? Perhaps the purpose of the journey is to feel the movement, see the passing away, and allow the gain to perceive evolution. So am I dying globally, physically, emotionally, or psychologically? Let me understand. What is happening? Let me see where I am going.

I had a week or two between the initial tests and the

results of follow-up tests to determine what type of tissue my body was making antibodies against. This is called ANA typing. We were also still waiting on some of the results from the first round of blood tests.

Purgatory: halfway between dead and alive while waiting for the judgment day. I see why our culture has deified physicians. Their opinions, dictates, and diagnoses are often the judgment we await. Am I sick? What is wrong with me? Will I live? What should I do?

Now, I'm a pretty independent sort. It occurred to me that if I wanted some voice in my destiny, I had better start answering some of these questions for myself and not give it all away. I guess I must have known this from the beginning. The first day I went to see Mary, I sat down in the upholstered chair opposite her desk and told her frankly, "I'm not interested in a diagnosis, really. I want to know what action to take. I am interested in moving through this place of illness. Whatever tests you think will help us know what to do, let's do them. I don't want a label. I want movement."

We never had to have that discussion again. Mary heard me, and set her mind and her heart on a track with mine.

I applied my intention and my attention to healing. Understanding was so important for me; I needed to comprehend what was happening— physiologically and spiritually. Like the miscarriage, it was likely to be part tragedy and part transformation. How can I find my way to the road of transformation? Through understanding the bigger picture and through surrendering again to the deeply held conviction that everything is as it should be. I couldn't just believe in God part time. My faith was being tested. This was no time to question divine will; it was time for making connections.

I had dedicated myself to the service of God, and I was well positioned for service. I had a well-established practice of bodywork. There was nothing that resonated with me about physical decline and disability, but if that wasn't the point, what was? An autoimmune disease meant my body was attacking itself. *I* was attacking *myself.* Something was happening under the surface of my conscious awareness; things were stirring deep within me. Intuitively, I knew that if I could understand where and how I was attacking myself, it may be my body would not have to play out the war for me. I had to change the outcome. I would need to avert war by making peace. I had some time before the next test results would come back. If I did my inner work, could I influence those results? It's just another example of field theory, so why back down? "Yes," I told myself, "I can."

The Tarot

John is a lovely man, an artist, a psychic, and a healer. He taught yoga for the ZB classes in Mexico each morning before breakfast. He skillfully sculpted his words with the principles of ZB and guided our bodies to experience these principles through poses and through breath. He also offered inspired Tarot-card readings. I had taken the opportunity to have him read a spread for me on two occasions. I had not thought of him much after our time in Mexico, but the audiotapes of those readings seemed to surface just when I needed to hear them again. The night before the rebirth ZB session in Connecticut, I drove from the class down to New Haven to have dinner with some friends. I chose a tape of my latest reading with John as I left home the day before, mostly because nothing else jumped into my hands as I was looking for music. I popped the tape in and laughed all the way down Interstate 91, wondering at how applicable the information was at this particular moment. Even though I understood and connected to it when he originally did the reading over a year earlier, it was as if it was meant to be heard on this day. We shared a laugh as he sat there, invisible in the front passenger's seat.

A few weeks later, while I was waiting for test results, this relative stranger and familiar spirit came back for another visit, but this time it was in my dreams.

I was walking in the woods when I met John standing at

the side of the path. We embraced in a hug that felt like home-by-the-fire after a day of skiing. No, it wasn't that cozy, it felt like letting someone hold my essence, like letting go, and like profound trust. I fell backward to the ground, which was now covered with snow and swept my arms and legs in and out to make a snow angel. In the snow, beneath the angel, I wrote, "I'm an angel!" He smiled. I looked down and at our feet there were many heart-shaped rocks. We looked at many of them, and then picked one that was perfectly shaped. Together, John and I placed the heart stone in the convergence of two trunks of the tree that stood in front of us. It felt like it was a key that unlocked something or a puzzle piece that, once in place, allowed the picture to be whole and visible.

It was immediately obvious that the timing of this dream was relevant to my current journey. I called John the next morning and left a message on his answering machine. I wasn't sure that he would remember me; we really had not had extensive interaction, although the connection was soulful. When he returned my call later that day, he assured me he did remember me. I told him about my dream, and he reminded me that when we last parted, he told me that I was an angel. He said he was quite serious and not attempting to flatter me or flirt with me. I remembered that sweet, clear, sincere good-bye vividly. The embrace in my dream had this same purposefulness that was not frilly, social, nor sexual. It was spiritual. We set up a time for another call when we could both spend an hour or so on for a Tarot reading.

Warm shafts of sunlight beamed through the double skylights in my office loft as I phoned John at the appointed time. After kind greetings, I quite literally asked him to put the cards on the table. I reviewed, for him, the events that led to this moment. I told him that I thought I was sick because I was stuck in separation. If I'm separate from myself, then one part of me can attack the other. I need to get back to one.

"I'm just not sure how to do that," I told him. "I'm waiting for a second round of test results, and I feel that I have this window of opportunity to come to a deeper understanding of the dynamics of all of this, to find out how to heal myself at the core of who I am. If I can find out how to mend my spirit, my body will not have to play out the drama for me."

John listened quietly and heard me completely. His voice was steady and grounding, "Well, let's see what the Tarot has to say."

He believes in his gift and easily lets the guidance of the Tarot flow through him. The sounds of fwopping and fwapping were decisive as he shuffled the deck and laid eleven cards on the table in a the form of a cross, with six cards on the horizontal axis and six on the vertical (the middle card is shared by both rows, so in this case six plus six equals eleven). "The vertical axis," he reminded me, "moving from the bottom to the top, generally represents what is in you from root to crown. The horizontal axis generally starts in the personal unconscious on the right and moves toward your conscious awareness as you go toward the middle, and then to how things are manifest for you in the external world on the far left."

He paused to consider the cards before him. "Tell me again, what is the connection between losing your hair and the ZB session in which you remembered the sadness at birth?"

"The hair loss is a symptom of the autoimmune condition," I said. "It is the clue that something is amiss. I connect the autoimmune condition to the belief system that I have apparently carried since birth that it is sad to be separated from God. So that must mean that deep within me I have the belief that being here in this body and in this life is not the right place for me. I am separate from my source here. So, maybe my body is finding a way to destroy itself to carry out a logical solution to a belief I didn't even know was there before that ZB session. I feel like I have one foot in heaven and one foot on earth. I'm literally being split down the middle. I feel paralyzed. It's making me sick. In my bones, I feel the experience of unity is possible. I can look around this beautiful blue-green planet and see the Garden of Eden, however, there is something that needs to change for me to embody that."

"Yup," John said confidently. "Okay. Just looking at this card spread briefly, just an overview of what I see is that you are very much in good shape. You are going through a phase of growth but deep down at the bottom of things, there's a shaky foundation. I think we'll find this relates to the kind of material that came up in that ZB session around birth. Do you feel that you fully dealt with the feeling of separation during that session?"

"I don't know that I dealt with it fully. I touched it,

felt it, and cried. But, I didn't have a long drawn-out process about it. In fact, right after I realized the sadness, I began to laugh uncontrollably. It struck me as incredibly funny that what I thought would be a fun evening trading ZB sessions and dining together became a profound rebirth experience. Tears of loneliness melted into tears of relief. I don't know if there is more there to deal with."

"Hmmm. Okay, well, starting with the horizontal axis of the card spread, with what is going on in the unconscious, we have the seven of cups. Cups are of the heart. Seven of cups appears when someone has an expectation of the heart that isn't met. This plugs right in to that session. It's really up in your unconscious, and it's there to be dealt with. You might want to get back to that material somehow. It shows up as you opening your heart and nothing comes back."

"Mmm-hmm."

"Since that's your first experience in life, it sets an undertone weaving itself through all aspects of your life. This is a fertile area to address. Now, I'm going to jump over to the vertical axis, at the bottom, because it shows the seven of swords, in the mind, as futility It's as if you are coming in, opening your heart, nothing happens, and your mind says, 'What's the use? I got off the bus at the wrong stop.' It's a feeling of bleakness."

It felt very important for me to hear the word *futility*. It was the right word for a very mysterious and unformed something I had felt tugging at me for as long as I could remember. I began to form an image of an anchor called futility sitting at the bottom of an immensely deep ocean, unseen and barely perceptible but definitely holding me back.

"Most of what I see in the rest of the spread," he continued, "is so in order, so aligned!"   With this underneath, it seems to me if you can really work through this shaky foundation, there is a lot of gain for you.   This will really bring a shift.   I am going to continue through the cards now and go back to the horizontal. The first card there was that seven of cups, the heart energy dishonored. Coming up to the level just below awareness, the second card on the horizontal, well, we actually have two cards because they wanted to be together when I put them down. They are the moon and strife. This tells me that some part of your energy had been tied up and unavailable to you because it feels like it won't be met and 'what's the use?'"

"Yes, it does feel like I've been keeping myself back."   The dark, dense, compressed sediment on the ocean floor began to stir and lift as the slack was taken out of the line. The anchor began to shift.

"Exactly, and that is diminishing your ability to move into your full self expression, which we see as we move along the horizontal to the position of awareness, and find the princess of cups.   She is a very, very beautiful being.   She is of the heart.   She is very spiritual.   In some decks she is shown under water, symbolizing surrender to God or to the Tao."

"Right."

"Now we are getting to the good news here.   It's like everything is in place, you just need to have all the energy going in the same direction at one time.   The

next cards on the
horizontal are science, truce, strength, and growth. You
are integrating deeply embodied knowledge—higher
knowledge from many lifetimes. As you come to peace
with both the personal and karmic picture of this
experience, you find your strength. The result is a major
step of soul growth that is bigger than this lifetime.

"You really do have a very valuable window of
opportunity. One which, I can tell you as a psychic, will
have a major impact on the rest of your life and future
lifetimes."

Fwop, fwop, fwop. I heard three more cards being
laid down.

"I am looking for a recommendation on *how* to deal
with this separation, and I didn't get at all what I might
have expected. So far, it doesn't say ZB or process
acupressure or another type of treatment. These three
cards tell me that you are moving into another phase of
your soul's development through many lifetimes. I see
change on the scale of eons. It brings tremendous
wealth, tremendous enrichment in the form of deeper joy
and happiness wherever you are. This process that you
are going through is literally shifting more than your
personal self and I am literally serious about you being
an angel, Michele. It's not flattery or anything like that.
One of the reasons you are here in this life is to help
alleviate the suffering in this world. You have—how
can I put this (and of course all of this is nothing for the
ego to get attached to)—but this is all much bigger than
yourself. In working through this separation thing, you
will be healing it for others. This is, quite frankly, the

first time I've seen this so clearly in maybe one thousand readings for people. You are working at a personal level and at a level of the collective unconscious because *you are an angel.* So, literally everything you do has more than a personal impact. Boy, that sounds like a big responsibility, but I didn't really mean it in that way."

"No," I mused, "I don't feel it that way. It feels kind of freeing, you know? Higher purpose is freeing."

"The fact that I didn't get what I was hoping for when I was looking for a recommendation on how to specifically work on this implies that you already know how. So, I'm going to go to the vertical axis, to the top card and tell you that you are crowned with victory!" he proclaimed playfully. The six of wands is up there. Magnificent! You have already won, and I can't imagine any way, at this point, that you could fail. If we come down below that victory to the position of the heart, we have the six of discs, which is called success. Below that, at the center of the spread, is again, the six of swords, science, which we saw on the horizontal as well. So you have three sixes, one over each other, and this is very beautiful because six, in the Tarot, is the number of greatest harmony and stability. It is the balance point between energy and structure! Sound familiar?"

"Hmmm. No wonder I love practicing Zero Balancing!" I laughed. Creating a balance between energy and structure is basically the definition of this unique and amazing work that brought John and I together in the first place.

"And if we go down to the belly," he continued, "at

the gut level, in the intuitive mind, you have the card called peace. This is a beautiful alignment here! But, at the base we have that futility because of the old bleakness that came in with the separation."

"That feels right. I get the image I am this cross you have laid out in the cards today, and the basic structure of who I am is strong and graceful. The floor is slippery, though and without a stable base, I can't quite gain a good reference point for success. I want to stop sliding around, so I can get a sense of where I stand and how to feel my strength. How can I see when my eyes are constantly pitching back and forth? I need to be still to orient my visual perception of my true self. Oh! And that relates to the vision thing. The ZB class where I had the rebirth session, I had been experimenting going without my glasses or lenses to see what I hadn't been able to see. I hadn't been seeing how pervasive this slippery surface of futility had been. I hadn't been seeing how the expectation of disappointment and loss had been sabotaging me. I have to mop up that floor somehow. That's my work."

"Absolutely," John agreed.

"Okay, so to recap," I wanted clarity, "I need to— what? Erase those early memories? I guess I don't really know how to do that. I don't know what it feels like to *not* have the futility and disappointment there. I *would* like to have another ZB session around it."

"Well, the cards did tell us you know how to do this, so maybe you should have more sessions around that until you really feel it is released. Over the next few years you'd probably notice all these shifts going on as it filtered down and rearranged things." He paused, and then added, "Do you have a spiritual practice?"

"I practice a kind of earth-based spirituality, based on a mixture of the cycles of the earth, sun, and moon, kind of superimposed on the Christian teachings of my youth. I am mystified by the teachings of animals, water, and plants. I've learned so much about the interface of heaven and earth just by studying the reflection of the world in rivers, lakes, and streams."

"Beautiful."

"Yes. It's magical. That's why I love this life, and why I love being in this body with its physical sensations. I love learning from nature. Like you said, the universe is in our field. I've learned that all teachings come to me if I remain open—there are the eyes, again. I open my eyes to the world and am willing to see things from innocence. That's my spiritual practice. I think of Zero Balancing as a spiritual practice, too. I have my hands at the interface of the physical and the spiritual nature of life every day when I work, and that is a practice of awareness. Touching energy and structure simultaneously and consciously is the practice of touching, seeing, and knowing the physical world while touching, feeling, and seeing the life force that animates it. One of my favorite quotes from Fritz is when he said he loves doing ZB because every time someone is on his table, he had the opportunity to touch God."

"Sounds like you've got what you need," John said confidently.

Clarity in Warts

Slowly over the next few days the point of my story was sharpened. If I was suspended in separation, if I was separate from myself, from God, and from spirit, then I could step away and look back at some part of myself. Further, I could turn on myself and attack myself. Why would I want to do that? Is my search for unity necessitating that half of my self dies? I don't want my physical body to have to die so my spirit can live. Maybe it is not the sword of Excalibur I need. Maybe it is the chalice—the Holy Grail. Can my spirit and my body come together in a deeper way than I currently know? Could they unite like the branches of the dream-time tree that formed a vessel in which John and I put the heart-shaped rock? I must heal the separation to heal my body. If there is unity, there is no other to attack. Can this resolve the expression of autoimmune disease? Perhaps disease is not a thing, but just dis-ease—a wrinkle that needs smoothing, a troubled soul on a ledge that needs to be talked down, or a situation teetering between resolution and collapse. It was an opportunity, a bifurcation, and a choice.

Knowing I needed to reprogram this early birth experience was not enough. I needed to *re-experience* the birth. Zero Balancing could help. I would go back to birth and experience something different and truer. I would be seen this time.

If one's life is dedicated to the service of God, God's authority cannot be questioned; there is only surrender to her will. If everything is God's will, then everything is exactly as it should be. If we offer no resistance to what is, everything is right. If everything is what is "supposed" to happen, whether painful, joyous, tragic, or comic, it is an opportunity and all events are laden with growth and light. When we become attached to something being wrong, we become guilty, victimized, or angry. The result, it seems, is arrested development.

Now there was a little more clarity on my path. I could go back to Mary's office and try to understand the data she had to share with me about my blood. Putting this together with the idea of unification, perhaps we could move forward. I was at peace. I felt magic return to my story. There was movement again.

****

A few days later, sitting in Mary's office, there were things I wanted her to say and things I didn't want her to say, but I didn't feel the clenching of anxiety in my chest. Having done some work to put the story in order, Mary's words would not be a judgment of what was wrong with me; they would be a tactical assessment that would help us formulate a road map to discovery—a you-are-here marker.

The ANA typing showed a speckled pattern that meant I was not making antibodies to my muscles or my heart, more likely to connective tissue. Connective tissue— issues of connection. Yes, yes. That's congruent, albeit still vague. We could do more testing, but Mary thought she would recommend the same course of treatment, whether we did or not. As she talked about liver function, my biochemistry-trained mind began to see the metabolic pathways churning. I found myself listening to her words from inside my own liver. Free radicals, cholesterol, and methyl groups rained down on me. I was being held captive by my own organ. My liver felt like a child who wasn't getting enough attention and was acting out to get what she needed. It was congested and dampened, arms crossed in defiance, and brow furrowed. I felt as though I needed to turn myself inside out, to sprout like a flower from the dark, moist soil of my body. I had germinated. It was time to grow.

Cells are born and die constantly, essentially forming new organs continuously. Some of the cells hanging out together today, forming my liver, may be dead tomorrow. New ones will take their place. Over days and weeks, all of the cells that make up my liver will have been replaced. With a significant change in our experience of ourselves, we have the opportunity to grow new and different organs as they are informed by the template of our larger self. If I am changing and being reborn, I may need a changed liver. Once again, I felt I had the bigger picture. It was all congruent.

As Mary began to write up what supplements she would suggest for our game plan, her officer manager, Suzan knocked softly at the door.

"Michele's blood minerals just came in," she said as she handed Mary a piece of paper.

"Oh, let's take a look," Mary replied

enthusiastically. She's always up for the challenge.

She only had to glance at the report. "Oh," she sang, quickly reformulating her plan. "Well, this could change things. Most of your blood minerals are very low, especially magnesium. The first thing we need to do is get you on some minerals. This could be the major piece. One of the cardinal signs of magnesium deficiency is rapid hair loss. We'll still work with your immune system, and we'll put you on minerals right away."

This was good news. I could do this. I could fertilize myself. I could eat more. I could eat better. I was so busy taking care of everyone else that I did not see I was neglecting myself. I felt a little foolish that someone needed to tell me this, but that was okay. Foolish is better than dead. Everything seemed lighter immediately. I felt as though I had taken a fork in the road or in the tree. I was now on the right path. I would stay true to my feelings and follow my heart toward healing. I would not give up my inner vision for the blind science of medicine. I would not forgo the inner journey for an external diagnosis. I would not forsake my faith in divine guidance for the judgment of any man. It was at the interface of vision and science, where the inner journey meets the outer course of action and my personal story aligned with my soul's quest that I would heal. My immune system would respond, and my liver would be rejuvenated and allow a new set of rules to govern my new life. I would feed the newborn me well and regularly. Hell, I knew how to be a good mom; I just needed to realize that *I* was the newborn.

****

But what about the ANA tests? What about the scientific proof that I had an autoimmune disease? How do I integrate that piece of information? I was not inclined to deny the test results, and at this point, I was no longer able to deny my own experience. I could only think of two possible explanations. Perhaps the ANA test was a false positive, and I was not actually making antibodies to myself. Or I did actually have antinuclear antibodies in my blood and had the genetic potential for the expression of an autoimmune disease, but I was learning how *not* to express it. Conscious evolution?

When there is a sudden change and it is perceived to be change for the worse, as with sudden illness, it is common to first look for evidence that it is not possible. There must be some mistake. When I first learned that I had a positive ANA test, I dove into my *Merck Manual of Medical Diagnoses*[9] to find an escape route. There, I did find that certain drugs, like aspirin, could result in a false-positive ANA test.

I had recently undergone treatment for a plantar wart on my heel. I had tried every natural remedy I could find to convince this belligerent colony of alien invaders to leave the premises, to no avail. Against my better judgment, I consulted a podiatrist. Not that I have anything against podiatrists, but I resisted the idea of having something cut off me without having come to balance of my own accord. However, when the wart grew be about an inch in diameter and was sending out scouts to establish satellite villages, I was frustrated, and I defaulted, like too many governments, to the unimaginative method of war to gain control. It was the virus or me. I felt intolerant and threatened by our coexistence. The podiatrist recommended burning the wart off with two different types of acid—a 30 percent solution of tricholacetic acid and a 40 percent solution of salicylic acid. We embarked on a campaign of weekly visits, so he could slash and scrape and burn the insurgents out of town. After each battle, he would dress the wound and send me off to let it smolder.

"Does this much acid have any systemic effect?" I asked. "I imagine it is absorbed through the skin."

"No," he said confidently. "There is no systemic effect. It just works locally."

But if the wound is bleeding when you put the acid on, what is keeping it from getting into my bloodstream and affecting other parts of my body? I thought to myself.

"Good," I said, completely giving away what I knew for the more palatable answer he offered.

I wanted to hear that there was no systemic response, so I accepted it. *He's the expert on these things, right?* Three weeks later, the night after the third acid application, I found it difficult to sleep. My heel was burning, my heart was racing, and I felt like I had five too many cups of coffee. I lay on the couch and did some deep breathing. After several anxious hours trying to fall asleep, I ripped the bandage off my foot. *This can't be good. I've had just about enough of this.* I cancelled my next appointment, and when my burnt skin healed, the triumphant colony was still flying its colors in the same one-inch circle on my heel. Two weeks later I began to notice my hair falling out.

Months later, faced with making sense of the test results, I learned that exposure to high doses of salicylic acid, which I had been wading in for weeks, can give a false-positive ANA test.

****

I had been visiting my chiropractor for spinal adjustments to support my whole system and relieve any stress on my nervous system that may have been contributing to the illness. The acid treatment had been abandoned months earlier, and the wart was as big as ever. Now that it was summer, I often kept a band-aid on my heel when I was barefoot; it was unsightly, possibly contagious, and embarrassing. Dr. Elizabeth noticed the band-aid and I told her what I had been through. She suggested I try methionine, an amino acid that supports liver function. She had some success using it for plantar warts with other patients; the theory being that there was a parasitic relationship between the virus that causes plantar warts and the host, so that the immune system was unable to identify the virus as alien and eradicate it.

Diving back into the *Merck Manual*, I learned that the wart viruses are circular double-stranded DNA, which enter the host's cells. If the wart virus had incorporated itself into my cells, perhaps my immune system was trying to deal with it by attacking the connective tissue of my own skin, trying to get at the DNA that was not me. Maybe I had headaches and fatigue because for years my liver was using up all its methionine ammo in the war of the wart. It was like Vietnam, fighting an enemy you can't see. Ahh, there's the connection to the eyes again. What can't I see?

The clues began to coalesce. Methionine is a methyl donor; it contributes little packages of carbon and hydrogen to the metabolic process called methylation in the

liver. Mary's plan to mediate the immune system by increasing my liver's ability to detoxify harmonized with this information from my chiropractor. The need for unification continued to be supported. I realized I must take up all of the space within my body and move the plantar virus out by displacing it with more of myself. I must come into myself more fully.

The biochemical piece was seen. I began to take methionine, magnesium, selenium, boron, vanadium, reduced glutathione, and antioxidants. I began to rebuild my body. Once the routine of eating regularly and taking my therapeutic doses of supplements was established, I could turn my attention to the energetic healing, to unification, to coming home to myself, and to being reborn in yet another way.

What I learned from the wart was that war doesn't work, and band-aids are not a solution. Healing means unification, and it happens, as chiropractors have been saying for over one hundred years, from above, down, and from inside, out. I had that plantar wart for over ten years and had tried every topical application known to treat it. When I learned I needed to claim all of the space within my body and nudge it out, when I started taking the supplements to support my bigger self, the virus shrank, the colonies evacuated obediently, and the wart completely and permanently disappeared within eight weeks.

Homeopathic Haircut

My fear of death and disease waned as the brilliant sphere of a co-creative world view rose on the horizon. I phoned my hairdresser and friend, Patti. I gave her the abbreviated version of the story and asked her if she would come to my house to cut my hair. After the Tarot reading with John, I had the distinct feeling the test results were being altered as my awareness of the healing process was expanding. I decided then, even if it turned out all of my hair wasn't going to fall out, I would cut it. I would make the statement to myself and to God that I got the picture. A homeopathic haircut: like cures like. I wanted it to be a ritual of release and gratitude for the outcome, for the turn around from disintegration to unification. Fortunately, we live in a small valley where the sense of community is strong. Patti and I had seen each other through many of the ups and downs of life, and she was right there for me. She was excited at the idea of using her skill in a ritualistic way and began to research the right short do for me.

****

I awoke feeling blue. Identified with loss, I allowed tears to flow freely down my cheeks. Dale had been constantly patient and supportive, but now his firm voice cut sharply through my self-absorption.

"It's only hair, for Christ sake. It could be a lot worse. What is the big deal?"

I know. I know. I must be so vain. Am I so identified with my appearance?

"It's just hard," I said.

"It will be okay, Shell," he replied softly. "I've always like women with short hair."

Hmmmm, I've had long hair since the day we met. "Oh, really? I had no idea," I laughed, lightening up a little.

While we waited for Patti to arrive, I lit candles and clarified my intention for this ritual.

I cut my hair in gratitude for my ability to see through the illusion of illness.

I cut my hair knowing that it will grow back stronger as I grow stronger.

I cut my hair homeopathically.

I release my attachment to my ego and to my appearance.

I acknowledge that the power to be fully who I am comes from within.

I am ready for change.

Dale's gentle scolding helped me to let go of the last bits of resistance. I was ready, and it felt good.

Patti bubbled through the front door, smiling and laughing as usual. She happily presented me with a clipping from a magazine showing me the haircut she recommended. The thing with my hair is that it curls in ringlets and has a mind of its own; I cannot have a style that requires control. My hair changes dramatically with the weather. If it's too short in the front, it will curl up tight in humid weather. It's like wearing a wool sweater that's been through the dryer. My friend Jenny once said to me, "Oh, you have a *fivehead.*" I looked at her quizzically, and she proceeded to explain that most people have foreheads, but some people have bigger foreheads, and they were known as fiveheads.

"We'll leave it a little longer on the sides and toward the front, and it will frame your face," Patti coached. She must have known about the fivehead thing, too.

I sat in a kitchen chair in my living room. Dale, the boys, and my friend and office manager, Denise gathered to watch. Patti suggested I make the first cut. Through a teary veil, I lopped off one big ringlet. The tears were for the beauty that alights when endings and beginnings speak to each other. It was as if the haircut was already completed on some other plane. Patti simply followed the plan and was done in no time.

I looked in the bathroom mirror and saw exactly who I had become. It was perfect. I loved the feeling of lightness and the softness of the small, feathery curls on my face. I was free. Patti and Denise fell into their own familiar connection and conversation. The boys ran off to play. Dale retreated to his shop. And I moved on.

****

I love to discover the sacred in the mundane. I love how the goddess presents herself in the dishwater, and how God appears during a car ride over the mountain to Brattleboro. Who would have thought that a haircut could become a fulcrum around which my journey would shift? It seemed that with each fork in the road new opportunities were presented. There seem to be places along the course of our lives where we can more easily jump from one lane to another, from one set of possibilities to another, and from one lifetime to a parallel one. One door was gently closed and another opened with the first clip of the scissors. It had happened in Mary's office as well. It was like the universe putting its turn signal on—you can change lanes now, if you like.

Each lane change was preceded by a feeling of detachment; I let go of the outcome and was in the present moment, allowing guidance to flow from where it will. Clinging to any particular or certain outcome would be resisting forward motion and the opening to fresh insight, either consciously or subconsciously. Meeting challenge with equanimity does not mean being disengaged. I was completely engaged in magic as I floated like an uncharged ion awaiting the next greatest potential to attract me and attune me to the quantum universe. Neither does it negate free will. If I am mostly space between tiny electron and protons, it is into the feeling of the freedom of that space that I must go before I can jump orbit. I am not only the physical particles of the electrons, I am the potential that they embody to move to new levels of excitement, to new orbits, new paths, new experience, and new outcomes.

But who ever heard of a homeopathic haircut? How does it work? I was experiencing an existence in which the unseen world of consciousness was primary. My physical form and life experiences became probabilities based on energy levels and electron excitation. The

nature of reality was dependant on how I moved my
energy. Access to endless possibilities seemed to relate
to how connected and responsive I was to my own
energetic state. Sometimes it was necessary to drive fast
and change lanes often, and other times to stay the
course. A flexible and adaptable energy body was as
much an asset as a strong and supple physical body.
Precision and grace on the journey through life was
relative to the ease of energetic interaction with the
somatic vehicle of my body and was reflected in a
dynamic interaction with the particular road I was
traveling.

Some great whole was trying to reveal itself. I
studied and learned many pieces from different fields of
study, but all trails led to the one great field: the
holograph of life. There is a bigger picture. It is bigger
than my human eyes can see. I need eyes and ears and
hands everywhere to know it. I cannot reduce it to know
it. The mystical Celtic poet, John O'Donohue speaks
eloquently of the soul's slippery nature in *Anam Cara*.
The soul, he says, does not like to be seen in the bright
midday sun. One must look at it kind of sideways, out
of the corner of the eyes, in the penumbral light of the
late afternoon.[10]   Quantum physicists claim that the
outcome of any event is immediately altered by the
presence of the observer. As soon as we see something,
it is changed. We cannot pinpoint a perception, we can
only flow with it and let it inform us of the whole.

Coyote Sells the House

Cutting my hair seemed to snip the ties that bound me to my past. Within a few days of the homeopathic haircut, Janet, our realtor called us with some hopeful news. Our house had been on the market for four long years with only an occasional interested looker. Janet thought she had someone who was seriously interested this time.

The Brown House is a great old house, but its location on Vermont Route 9 was not favorable for many perspective buyers. Buyers interested in commercial property found it was just a few houses too far out of the village and had limited parking. For those interested in a residence, there were quieter places.

She was a true Vermonter of an old home with nooks and lofts and secret passageways, alluring in her charm, but a quagmire in terms of energy movement. There were doors that went nowhere, doors that only went somewhere if you were thin enough, and doors that did not close properly. The stairs were narrow and steep. There were many acute, often incongruous angles marking the threshold of successive ownership. She had mellowed over the years with a signature of creativity, love, and appreciation in her timbers, but had become a little scattered in her old age. Perched above Main Street, her eyes constantly tracking the coming and going of the world, she was getting tired. Sills had rotted in a few spots, and beams were bowing. Each winter, a few more slate shingles cracked under the glacial ice jams on the roof and fell like loose teeth from her brave smile. The Brown House grew old with the soft furrowed face and welcoming lap of a loving, wise, and accepting grandmother.

Each night, when I would snuggle the boys into bed in the Brown House, we would pray "Thank you, God, for another beautiful day on earth. Thank you for our beautiful family and for our healthy bodies. Thank you for all of our abundance, for our food and clothes, and our beautiful house that keeps us warm and dry. Thank you for the land. We hope there is a family that wants to buy our house, so we can build a new house and live at the land. We know the new family will benefit from all the good energy, love, and happiness we have found in this house." Any additional thank you comments that were appropriate to the day were added, and then we would send the prayer off with: "Thank you for being in the grace of God. Amen."

Our prayers are always answered, of course, although not always in the manner we expect. This time Great Spirit sent his old friend Coyote with the answer. Coyote is the trickster and brings his medicine upside down. Crazy, inside-out lessons that turn over the apple cart but then teach you the delight of apple pie. Coyote entered the temple of my ancient body, invaded grandmother's house and was turning things upside down. He was turning my cells against me. He locked my grandmother up in the closet and put on her clothes. Ah, but she had already taught me to be steadfast and brave. She continued to tap, tap, tap Morse code on the closet door. "Do not believe the coyote. You are whole. He is not your ancestor. Keep moving. Keep looking." With her encouragement, I looked the coyote in his yellow eyes, and he went running up the back hill. I released grandmother from the closet, and she released me from her tutelage. "Go," she said. "You are ready. Build your own house now."

When Janet brought the perspective buyer and her realtor by to see the house, I knew they were the family we had prayed for. Melissa was a young single mother with four small daughters. The spirit of the Brown House seemed to fold them into her skirts immediately and say, "Yes." Melissa said yes, too. We agreed to move out in three weeks.

Turn, Turn, Turn

It was spring of the year 2000, and the winds of divine orchestration were blowing. My body was reorganizing and some walls had to be torn down for the expansion project. It is said that when houses appear in our dreams, it is often symbolic of our bodies. In many traditions mystical journeys are described as a coming home. So, for me, selling our house at this time of rebirth and reorganization made perfect sense. It was time for a turnaround in my body and a turnaround in my home. The Byrds' 1965 ecclesiastical folk rock classic became a daily mantra:

> To everything, turn, turn, turn
> There is a season, Turn, turn, turn,
> And a time to every purpose
> under   heaven.[11]

It took a lot of reflection to find the flow. Deep in my bones I knew I had much work to do in this life. I was born to teach, and I hadn't even begun that work yet. The image of the bifurcation in the tree trunk from my dream was ever present. The two paths diverging in the woods from Robert Frost's poem "The Road Not Taken" lay before me.[12] The path to the left was wider and flatter and the horizon more visible. The path to the right was overgrown and grassy, and it dove into the mystery of the woods. To the left was diagnosis and identification with limitation, with the not so rightness of me.   To the right was unknown, but free.   Faith slipped under my right foot, trust guided me to the path less traveled, and ironically, that has, indeed, made all the difference.

As I understand it, hair, in Chinese medicine, is related to the kidneys, to the bone, to water, to deep ancestral patterns, and to the energy of conception. With the haircut, there was a release of old, ancient ancestral patterns; a letting go of an old way of being.   It seemed that as I loosened my grasp on who I thought I was, the walls of our old house could release us.

A chaos similar to the one I had just encountered in my body shook my home as well.   We had lived in the Brown House for ten years.   Ten years of the residue from our lives had to be sorted, packed, cleaned, and scraped from closets, drawers, cabinets, walls, floors, stairs, and ceilings.   I would have cleaned out closets and cabinets more regularly if I had someplace to unload unused and outdated things.   I disliked the idea of bringing toys and appliances to the dump to be buried in the precious earth.   With three weeks to vacate, I was clearing things in any way that I could.   We had a large dumpster   delivered   and   filled   it   to   overflowing. Somehow, being just one dumpster, albeit a very big one, it seemed less offensive than bag after bag, trip after trip, to the dump.   By this time there was a great second hand shop in town called Twice Blessed.   They took in used clothes and household items to sell them at very affordable prices, using some of the profits to help community families in need.   I brought old toasters, mixers, cookware, and clothes to be reused.   We had a yard sale. I sold my couch and matching chair for $40 to an incredulous and elated young mother. That was fun. We sold and gave away books, toys, clothes, furniture, antiques, and knick-knacks. No more knick-knacks.

Simultaneously, we began to search for a rental house and an office for my practice. After looking at a few places that may have been sufficient, if not homey, Mary Beth, my new office manager offered one of her fulcrums.

"How about Dotty and Kevin's place? It's empty, and I don't think they come up much anymore." She was referring to a charming old farmhouse less than a mile down the road that had been vacant for a year or so since the owners had moved to New York. "You could probably even use the front two rooms for a temporary office. There's a separate entrance, and a bathroom, and there's plenty of parking."

I could immediately see my children exploring the stream that skirted the property and jumping in the pond behind the house, although I had my doubts about whether the owners would want the public coming and going in a house that they were trying to sell.

"Are they renting?" I asked.

"No. But they might."

I called Kevin in New York that night. After a brief discussion, he said he would certainly consider the idea. He would talk it over with his wife. I didn't mention the part about the office. I wanted him to like the idea of renting first, and then I would mention commercial use. He called back the next day.

"I talked it over with Dotty," he said, "and we think it would be fine. You know, you could probably even use the front two rooms as your office. There's a bathroom there, and the front door could be a separate entrance, and there's plenty of parking."

Done deal. The universe just kept saying yes.

White Mountains

Soon after moving into the farm house, I was invited to chaperone a backpacking trip in the White Mountains of New Hampshire with the High School Leadership Program. My friends, Joellen and Bob, were coordinating the program, which trains high school students in leadership and communication skills with the goal of preventing drug and alcohol abuse. Jo and Bob wanted to share their love of the outdoors and the challenges of backpacking with the group. Because of a conflicting beach party, several students backed out of the trip, and we ended up with a lovely mix of six young women and six adults. Having no daughters, I was delighted to spend three days in the mountains with teenage girls.

Ascending Mount Washington on the Ammonoosuc Trail, we climbed three miles and rose 2,400 vertical feet. We witnessed each other move through the challenges of the journey, encouraging each other when burdened shoulders burned and rubber legs wobbled. It was heartwarming to see how, with kind words of support and trail mix with M&Ms, we kept each other going.

When we arrived at Lake of the Clouds hut, we enjoyed a warm dinner prepared by young adults, mostly college students on their summer break. Lake of the Clouds is one of the largest of the high huts, sleeping ninety people in eight jam-packed bunk rooms. I was truly inspired by our hosts and hoped that my sons would reach for such experiences someday. They welcomed and organized hikers, cooked and served two meals a day, and packed in all the supplies on their backs weekly. When tired hikers were snoring in their bunks, the "croo" would seek out nocturnal adventures. Raids have been a part of hut life for decades. Under the cloak of darkness, they would hike five miles or so to another hut and confiscate some prized possession that had likely been borrowed from their own hut many times over. The night we were there, they hiked to Lonesome Lake hut and reclaimed an eight-foot steel propeller that had been scavenged years ago from the wreckage of a plane crash. It must have weighed a few hundred pounds, and they carried it all the way back up the trail that we labored over with our slight forty-pound packs! I fell in love with their lives, with their strength, and with their spirit.

All night, as the crew pilfered and as I slept, my thoughts were organizing themselves with a kindred passion. I awoke before dawn, probably about the time the crew members were returning from their mission, although all was quiet. I fumbled for my flashlight. It was 5:15 A.M. Ideas were coalescing and presenting themselves to my consciousness with wild abandon. Perhaps it was the elevation, near the peak of the highest mountain on the East Coast that inspired this unusual clarity. Hoping that my hand would know how to put the words down in a comprehensible order, I opened my journal and poised my pen. My awareness was amplified. The mountain was offering me a clearer, stronger field. I felt transparent. The story in my bones pulled me in. I surrendered to my own mission and to places in my body I never knew I could access. I posed the question *why am I making antibodies to myself?* Suddenly, I found myself sliding through my bloodstream, wriggling my way across cell membranes, shoving proteins and fatty acids aside, and swimming through cytoplasm to come face to face with my nuclei. My nuclei? Why would I be making antibodies to my nuclei? I slipped through the membranous wall of a nucleus and witnessed my DNA unzipping. I wrote:

My DNA is unzipping. I'm unraveling. I've become undone. I'm separating. That's the key. Everything is tumbling into place, perched here on top of the White Mountains, as the earth tumbles toward a new day. I'm unzipping because I'm separated. Flashing back to the events of the past few years, I could see how the old me had become undone and the new me was being synthesized. DNA actually does unwind, exposing its underbelly, as it replicates itself. What are the events? I asked to be in the service of God in a ZB session in Mexico because that was the core of it all. The only thing left to do was surrender to a higher power to move with optimal grace through this mystery of life. As the day dawns, I can see that I still believed God was other than me. God was still in some way a guy in the sky, away from me, and I was a lowly servant. While this humility serves me in surrender, part of this life view does not serve. Separation from the divine does not serve me. It make me feel alone and empty.

I take off my glasses and ask to see what I am not seeing. I receive another ZB session, and I see my own birth. I am alone there, too. No one is looking in my eyes. No one sees the God in me. I can't see God. I am separated from my source. I am so sad. Then, I am sick, and I am tired—tired of treading water. I need someone to hold me. My head aches, my hair is falling out. I am almost all unzipped.

Here, on top of the visible earth, I saw what it meant to be suspended in the vibration of separation. There was a void in my field, and I was striving, working, straining, and dying for connection. My cells were doing just what they were supposed to do. Immune cells are designed to attack foreign invaders, and I had been subconsciously giving my cells the command of disintegration. I had declared war on the part of myself that didn't belong in this world. I continued to allow insight to flow from the tip of my pen:

In the stillness of the day's first light there is peace. I know what I have to do to heal. I see the ever-growing picture from my mountain perch. I am not only closer to God up here surrounded by beauty and light, I am God, I am beauty, and I am light. I have to get it together. I must refocus on my wholeness, on my connection to my source. I am being reborn, and there is a potent opportunity to reset the vibration, to reorganize the ground substance of how I am in the world. Having traveled into my cells, I can see who I am and what I need, though I can't completely hold the feeling yet. I must reach deeper into myself, below my conscious awareness, into the matrix of my bones to reprogram the core experience of separation. I must accept unity in my

DNA.

I was amazed at the clarity that came in my writing, and that clarity brought more questions. I had been taught that DNA holds the genetic blueprint of who we are. How did the blueprint, the energetic imprint get in our DNA? And if my DNA was unzipping, what was changing? What did I inherit and what no longer serves me? My heavy head leaned on my forearm, and I slipped into a half-awake dream.

As the fog lifts from behind my eyes, I can see a woman from another time. It is both me and my mother's mother's mother. We are one. She is thin, worn, and tired. She wears a faded floral dress and a once-white apron. Standing in a field, picking through the soil, she is trying to harvest enough crop for her family. Her hands are rough, knobby, and raw. She has literally worked her fingers to the bone. The potatoes are rotten. There is not enough, and there will never be enough, she thinks. Her gaze is distant and empty as she looks out over the fields. She is looking for me, her survival. She bends to the earth and works on because that is all she can do. It is Ireland during the potato famine. It is now. I feel her sadness and futility. Her DNA is vibrating within me. The frequency of poverty has moved through my whole life. The rug will always be pulled out from under me. I can plant the crops, work 'til my hands bleed, but there will not be enough. There is the shaky foundation. God is there but inaccessible. I got off the bus at the wrong stop.

If I can see her, can she see me? Can I help to heal her life by being the highest expression of me? Is she doing her work, so that I can do mine? I feel a loving duty to evolve for her. She doesn't need me to carry her vibration; she needs me to carry mine. She can feel me and I give her hope. I can feel her and she is my root. I will sprout and flower for her.

Knowing the Void

Naked DNA—unzipped and exposed. Now I can see
dimensions of myself I have not seen before. This
slippery surface of ground substance goes further back
than my birth. The void that seems to have been woven
into the fabric of my being has been programmed into my
ancestors for generations. Separation and poverty are
only a nuance apart; both could be defined as
disconnection from nourishment, from that which
sustains. The deep loss has been part of my background
field. I have inherited it along with my Irish face. Can it
be a specific gene, a sequence of nucleic acids that tells
our cells what peptides and proteins to synthesize? Is
there a poverty protein? Antibodies are proteins. Perhaps
the antinuclear antibody is the poverty protein, or is the
expression of my underlying belief in loss and futility
more related to the cadence, the vibration, the rhythm of
my DNA, than to the structure alone?

When my DNA unzips, I come across the hidden
song of poverty and loss. What does it look like? I can't
see it, and it isn't a sound; it's the space between sounds.
It is the cessation of the rhythm of life; it is an absence
without end, and it is so big that I begin to fall into it. Has
my subconscious buried this feeling away from me so that
I would not have to feel the root deep in my pelvic floor
pulling out of the soil of this life?

Perhaps this vast, depressed space in my genetic code
leads to my fear of heights. My DNA resonates with the
void, and I begin to fall into it while I'm still six feet from

Which is what I have been doing all day.
Tell me, what else should I have done?
Doesn't everything die at last, and too
soon?
Tell me, what is it you plan to do
With your one wild and precious life?[13]

A challenge from the grasshopper:

*What will I do with this one wild and precious life?
I will be seen, I will be held, and I will connect with the
divine nature of this world.*

Friday night rolled around. Jim and I sat side by
side on a ZB table in the large meeting room where class
was held. A student had asked to observe the session
and sat quietly off to the side.

"So, how can I help you with this session?" Jim
opened.

"I've been working on reprogramming my DNA. I
am turning off the separation/autoimmune gene I
became aware of in the ZB when I remembered my
birth. I would like to go back to that birth place and
imprint something different. I would like to experience
being met, being held, and being seen. I would like to
be welcomed into this life, into this body, and I would
like to be unified instead of separated."

He probably asked a few more questions to clarify
my intention—the frame for my ZB session—for
himself and for me. Lying on my back on the table, I
surrendered to the process of the session, allowing the
evaluation and observing the effects of balance. A mini-

dream transported me from waking consciousness to a
state of altered consciousness:

*I am standing on the curb. I feel I need to go on a
healing journey. Looking out in to the maze of city
streets, I don't know which way to turn, but I know there
is a bus station behind me. I spin around and enter
through the revolving door. There is an authoritative
looking man behind the counter. I tell him I am ill and
need to go on a journey to reclaim my health. I tell him
I would like to turn off a gene, alter the rhythm of my
DNA, and be reborn into unity.*

*"Can't be done," he says. "But we can help you.
Sit here with your illness. I can tell you exactly what it
is called. You don't need to go anywhere. Have a cup of
tea, some steroids, and a couple of Prozac."*

*Unsatisfied, I look around. There is an
experienced-looking woman behind another counter.
She listens to me for a long time. She asks many
questions. When she is satisfied that she understands
me, she makes a plan.*

*"Here are your bus tokens. You will need these to
ride the bus. Here is your lunch. You will need to eat
during the ride. Here is a map to where you want to go.
There are several bus routes that could take you there,
and you can choose among them—just keep going
toward your destination. I'd like you to check in with
me along the way, so we can make sure you get there
safely. Go out to the curb and choose a bus to begin
your journey."*

*Back out on the street, there is already a bus at the
dock. The placard reads ZB. Oh, I've taken this bus*

before. I like this bus—smooth ride and good drivers. I'm on board.

I knew that Zero Balancing could move me through my autoimmune condition more than any medical testing or procedure. I was not critical of the medical field; without the diagnostic understanding of this situation, I would not have been able to put the whole story together. But, there are places, deep in the healing process, where western medicine does not go, and I needed to go there. So, I asked, in framing my session, for some things that to the inexperienced ear, may sound unattainable through a bodywork session. I had no doubt Jim would have little difficulty taking me there. He's an excellent driver.

The session appeared very subtle. I was only aware of the student who was observing a few times, when I thought to myself, *"I wonder what his experience is? Can he tell what I am feeling?"* I'm not sure *I* was even aware of what was shifting for most of the session. There was no thunder and lightning or emotional catharsis. I felt deeply relaxed, cared for, and very trusting. I was not thinking about DNA or separation or rebirth. I was enjoying the sensations of energy moving in my body: relaxation, flow, warmth, comfort, and surrender. I didn't have to think.

There was one particularly memorable fulcrum near the end of the session. Jim asked if there was anything else he could do in the session before he finished. I checked in with myself. I felt great. I felt met, held, and seen on many levels.

"No, there's nothing else."

There was a pause. There are lots of pauses in ZB sessions—time to integrate, reflect, feel, and organize. I felt satisfaction with the session and simultaneously felt that there *was* something else I wanted. I wanted my very heart to be touched and to be seen. I wanted all of the beauty and magic I knew in this life to be witnessed. I said nothing. It's very intimate—touching hearts, and I didn't want to have to ask Jim to go there with me. It's a tender place; maybe it's a solitary place, I thought.

I knew Jim was aware that I was still processing whether I could/would/should ask for anything else. As he was finishing the session, he stood at the side of the table listening with his whole self. And then he took my hand. This was not in the protocol. It was a creative response to my unspoken desire. He was holding my hand. It was so sweet and gentle and welcoming. I knew then, I could have everything I wanted. On one hand I did not want to cross the line of too much intimacy with my revered teacher, but on the other, I knew he could hold it. I took his hand and placed it over my heart, silently asking him to witness all that I am and all that I feel. It felt good. After a moment, he placed *my* hand where his had been and placed his hand on top. *Was he trying to remove himself a little? Was it too much? Never be too much*—the old limitation that I had learned somewhere and too many times spoke to me. *Never be too much.*

Well, now or never, I thought. *Be too much,* I told myself. *Be everything. Feel everything. Connect to everything.* I left my hand on my heart and put my other hand on top of his. And it was okay. My eyes were still closed. I smiled so wide and real. I was home.

I took my time getting off the table, or more accurately, time took me. I felt delightfully heavy, as if my electric charge had been restored and now the magnetic field of the planet had something to grab on to. Talk about being held. The metallic core of the earth was gathering me up like a mother clutches an injured child to her breast. Sometimes clients feel a significant change or release in the middle of a ZB session and sometimes the awareness of the shift comes at the end or even after the session is over. A session is complete when the client is up and walking on her own legs, reorienting to the world in the upright position. As I tried to maneuver in this new relationship with gravity, my left leg made its way to the edge of the table and slid off the side. I lay that way for a minute, maybe two, but it felt like ten. Finally, my right leg joined my left, and I sat up. Once seated, it was relatively easy to stand and walk, and thank my practitioner and my witness for a great session.

We all walked outside, where we were greeted by the rising moon and a party of mythological characters dancing in the night sky. We stood in silence, stunned by the beauty of the night. I had no words. Something was changing in the fabric of my being, and I couldn't quite find my reference point. Feeling the need for self-observation, I excused myself. I walked slowly across the yard to my room, put on my bathing suit, and went back out under the curious night sky to bask in the hot tub alone. The moon and the stars were my witnesses now; they put their collective arms around me and held silent council with my soul.

The next morning, during a break, Jim asked how I was doing. I didn't really know until that moment what I was experiencing, but I earnestly wanted to share my experience with this man who had been there for me since my first footsteps into the world of ZB. I closed my eyes, checked in with myself, and heard my voice saying, "I feel as if all the molecules in the universe have substance. Like there's this matrix that is holding me within it. I used to feel like being here was treading water in a vacuum, and now there is this lovely palpable mass to the space around me. The universe is holding me. I'm one with the universe."

I didn't need to have the same dreamlike vision of my actual birth. I didn't go back and remake the movie, coercing the characters' limbs into a more acceptable embrace. I wanted to be held. Beheld? The gentle fulcrums of ZB loosened the fibers in the material of my world view, and the old beliefs were lifted out like stains in a laundry detergent advertisement. I saw myself and allowed all of myself to be seen. I was reborn into a new way of being in the world.

Unzipping Geese

Haying season has come and gone; tractors and mowers are settled in barns and sheds for the winter. The October sky is gray. Fields are thick with long-neglected grass, soggy and stiff with the autumn frost, as Kayla and I set out for an early morning hike. We head for the trail that loops behind the rented farmhouse, up the northern hill, overlooking the village. Walks in the woods are always a journey into someplace deeper. With Kayla, this almost always involves some discovery. It may be a natural wonder like a cave scattered with porcupine quills or a broadened understanding of ourselves and our relationships. Usually it's both.

We skirt the pond and cross the inlet stream on a little wooden bridge. Winding along a quiet path cushioned by moss and decaying leaves, we speak of the circumstances of the day, of our coming together, and of gratitude for waterproof hiking boots. The trail emerges from under the canopy of trees and opens to a steep, grassy hill. Kayla and I weave deeper in to our stories as our breaths expand and our strides lengthen. Our legs burn with the uphill push. Emotion is lifted from the freshly oxygenated places in our tissues; we speak of the frustrations and gratitude of finding time for ourselves. We clear our bodies and minds, moving through the emotional layer, until, at the top of the hill, we pause to catch our breath under the calm eye of a solitary white pine. We look out over the Deerfield Valley, where autumn fire and flourish have receded to the duller hues of what we call "stick season." The skeleton of the land emerges. Where trees once wrapped us in a fleecy blanket of color, now there are stark vertical trunks and bare gray limbs. Soft breezy kisses are replaced by nipping bites on roughened cheeks. The glass grass crackles underfoot. I feel a little less held by the natural world and more exposed to it. My eyes focus on more distant horizons, but I feel more vertical. It's as if God can see into the top of my head without the sheltering New England canopy.

We continue on our path, passing through an opening in a stone wall. If the deciduous trees are the seasonal dress of the landscape, stone walls are the ageless skeletons. The organically linear walls of rock, too committed for the icy hands of winter to move, are held together by the dreams and sweat and prayers of the people who have loved this land for generations. They are all the more beautiful for the springy green moss and irresistible, sweet, vibrant lichen that feed on their demise. They carry a secret code of evolution from the stewards of the land before us.

Kayla and I are resonating with the land and with each other, for now that we are within the sacred walls of what I call the Middle Meadow, the space between us becomes highly charged and silent. There are ancient, unseen things here, peeking out from behind prehistoric rocks dropped by glaciers during their not-so-hasty retreat. Eons ago, this meadow offered the giant ice arms a place to rest their burden, as it does for us today. It offers a place to put down the business of everyday living and descend into deeper listening. It is a transition place, a misty place between worlds, and a threshold where the veil thins. The Middle Meadow is a place where the elements are as curious about us as we are about them. They watch and follow and tease us. Knowing how much we would love to catch a glimpse of some physical form, some structure, they mischievously offer only a breeze, a rustle, or a wink in the air. Having walked here many times, I know that if I stop and wait and study and strain for something more, it just becomes more still and silent. It's a slippery place; the offering here is the dance itself, the feeling of magic that opens one's consciousness to something else. If there were a signpost here it would read Listen Deeply. And when you passed the sign and turned around, on the back it would read Keep Moving.

Like a perfectly placed fulcrum, Kayla asks, "So how are you doing, Shell? Tell me what you know about your body and how you are healing. You've said something about DNA. What's going on there?"

We haven't had an opportunity to talk for any length of time since the summer backpacking trip to Mt. Washington. As we move purposefully through the meadow, I slow down and drop into intimacy, into myself. My words come slowly at first, as my awareness shifts gear.

"I think that I have reprogrammed my DNA." I had not yet spoken of these thoughts, visions, and revelations in any linear way. It comes in bits and pieces.

"Can you tell me more about how that happens?"

As she sees me descending into the inner vault of my intellect, she realizes she is in for a lesson and a story. Her eyes sparkle and widen like a child sitting on her grandmother's lap. She squeezes my arm with her two hands. "Tell me about DNA! How does it work?" she squeals. Kayla has an endearing way of pulling the truth from my bones. I often don't know what it is I have to say until she interrogates me. She interviews me. She would make a masterful talk show hostess. Now she is pulling this biology lesson from wherever it has lodged in my mind.

"Well, you know DNA is a double helix, like a spiral, right?" I ask as I model the spiral with my forearms.

"Like eagle pose," we say simultaneously, laughing. Kayla is my yoga teacher, and we have the precious opportunity to weave lessons from our chosen fields of study into the continuous tapestry of understanding and friendship. Eagle pose is a yoga position where the forearms and legs are spiraled around each other.

"DNA holds our genes," I continue. "Genes are encoded segments of DNA. The sequence of molecules, called bases, along the DNA strand determines our genetic makeup. Particular sequences of these bases are responsible for the synthesis of specific proteins. Proteins serve as enzymes, which help keep all the chemical reactions in the body working smoothly, and proteins also form the structure of our bodies, like muscles, bones, skin, and hair. DNA is like the blueprint holding the plan for what we are made out of, what our structure is, and how to make that structure work in the world. We inherit this genetic material from our parents and from our ancestors. Most people believe what is in our genes is in our genes and that's just all there is to it. What I'm feeling, however, what this illness has shown me, is that genes can be turned on or off based on our *experiences*. We can have a gene our whole life, but it can be dormant. There is such a thing as gene expression, a state in which certain genes are turned on for some unknown reason. For example, it's common for degenerative autoimmune diseases to be expressed genetically around the age of forty, especially in women, but we don't really know why."

The lesson pauses here so Kayla and I can negotiate the crossing of a little stream that carves a shallow depression at the edge of the meadow. We crouch down and cup our ears, listening to the drumbeat at the heart of the stream. Crossing this threshold, we begin to climb through a small stretch of maples to the upper meadow.

"So," I continue, "I think our experiences, our energetic dynamics can turn on and off our genes. Our thoughts, beliefs, and reactions create certain frequencies of energy, certain vibrations, which affect our genes."

I let that thought settle while observing our breath, which has become deep and steady, is now synchronized like two drummers playing together. Did the stream do that?   Not interested in stopping the dance, Kayla observes the rhythm and picks up the melody again.

"Okay, so how would that happen? How do we turn genes on or off?" she asks as she leans into me.

"Well, for example, I had experienced separation in various emotionally charged ways. First, I experienced the deep grief of separation from my baby, and within that I perceived a separation from the divine hand of God. Then I had that ZB session where I remembered my birth and the experience of being separated from my mother and simultaneously being separate from the rest of life—being alone. Looking back from where I am now, there were many other manifestations of the energy of separation that I have been living with my whole life. I struggled with the consciousness of poverty. Always, beneath the surface there was the belief that the rug was just about to be pulled from underneath my feet, and I'd lose what I had. I felt separate from the source of my life, my nourishment, and separate from the great mother."

We pass though the opening in another stone wall and the trail ends at the suggestion of a grassy hill. There is no choice; we are called onward to the top, to the destination, where the journey would turn us toward home again.

"In my experience, the layers of separation kept coming, one wave upon another, becoming amplified in my consciousness. These waves crashed down all the doors keeping me away from the sorrow of the original archetypical separation from God. The realization of loss and sorrow actually opened the doors within my cells, flooded through the structural fortress of my cell walls, and cascaded right into the core of my being. The nucleus is like a cell within a cell, and the DNA, the blueprint, is within the nucleus. The waves kept coming and not only broke through into the nucleus but broke into the DNA itself.

It sounds very mechanical, but I think the mechanism is vibrational in nature. Receptors on cell surfaces can change vibrational states. When they do, they effect movement across cell membranes, movement of particles like sodium, potassium, and proteins that are importing and exporting information. Science has been looking far too long only at the *particles* and missing the connection to the *information* they carry. We don't know how to measure that information, and it is not as controllable as the particle itself. The life energy accompanies the particles. Our cells are changed by the information exchanged—by the feelings, emotions, thoughts, and beliefs that move within them and between them. Our minds are not located in our brains. Our emotions are mediated throughout all the cells of our bodies. So, our experiences can get right into our cells and into our DNA. My life circumstances opened up the feeling of sorrow, revealed the belief in separation, resonated with the ancient sorrow and separation already programmed into my DNA through my ancestry, and caused it to unzip. The strands are unwound in some way, exposing the code within."

As if on cue, a penetrating north wind begins to push at our backs, lifting our bones, as we trudge up the hill toward Meditation Rock, the highest and most exposed point of our hike.

Meditation Rock was named by Justin, when he was four-years-old. We would hike up there from the Brown House. It was our resting spot; I would bring a snack for Justin, so he would be happily occupied while I listened to the voice of the north wind coming over Haystack Mountain in the distance. Meditation Rock was the place where we both learned to trust what we heard from the earth.

"Tell me about the unzipping! How does DNA unzip?" Kayla has a playful innocence when it comes to digging out information. She's like a puppy, never wanting to stop chasing the ball.

A sharp OH-AAH-GH comes in answer but not from me. We look up to see an uncharacteristically disorganized flock of Canada geese making their way toward warmer weather. Apparently OH-AAH-GH means WATCH. Geese have a way of moving, always rearranging and reorganizing, which is mesmerizing. As we give the geese our attention, they organize, not just themselves, but all the molecules of air between them and us. They reach us. We are with them. All other sensory input from the environment is externalized. We are connected to their matrix. Gracefully and efficiently they form two parallel lines out of their apparent disarray. They move as if in slow motion, wings whirring as feathers are pulled through the air. To our utter delight and amazement, the two lines of birds veer toward each other and, one bird at a time, spiral around each other then separate into two distinct lines again. As they continue southward across the sky, the two lines of geese zip back together to become one long, unified vector. It was a spontaneous half-time show.

"Oh, my God."

"Oh, my goddess."

We stand in silence, faces uplifted to the light, until they pass out of sight. When we turn our faces to each other, our eyes are wide, and mouths still open. We squeal like little girls and embrace each other, jumping up and down.

"Thank you!" I call after them.

Bringing It All Together

Just because geese speak to us does not mean Kayla is about to put the ball down.

"What else can you tell me about DNA?"

"Well, I can tell you what I think, and what I experience. When our DNA is touched by the energy of our experiences, it has the opportunity to shift or change. I don't know how it all happens. That's up to researchers to figure out, I guess. I just know what I experience.

Perhaps the frequencies of thoughts, beliefs, and feelings resonate with the frequency at which our DNA or some part of it vibrates. We might call that resonation the *ring of truth*. When DNA unwinds, exposing its inner code to its partner RNA, and if a particular vibrational state is present, genes in the DNA can be moved into an excited state and turned on, or they can be quieted and lulled to sleep.

If turned on (expressed), the sequence of molecules that make up the gene will make certain proteins, and those proteins will have a specific job to do. They'll go about doing their job until the circumstances are aligned for that gene to be quieted (not expressed). In me, the vibration of separation turned on a gene responsible for making antibodies that attack the material in my own cells. It is called an antinuclear antibody or ANA.

It makes sense, really. If I am experiencing myself as separate from my source, then I am other than myself. I am two selves—the divine self and the mortal self. It's the ultimate illusion. There is not room in this body for both of us, and one of me must destroy the other. That is the function of the immune system—to identify and destroy whatever is alien.   I figure God is not going to lose, so either my mortal self has to die, or I have to come together in one self. I'm choosing the later. It will be more pleasant for everyone.   I have to heal the separation at my core, to replace that story with another one. And that *is* my story."

We are still standing on Meditation Rock. Kayla's long legs are planted in a wide stance, her intense eyes are fixed on mine, and her teeth are dug into a mission of understanding.

"How do you do that? How do you heal the separation, Shell?"

I told her about my last ZB session at Angel's Rest.

"It's so wild! The whole Eden thing—this healing journey has been orchestrated by the birth of Eden, the spirit who is waking me up to the essence of the Garden of Eden. I'm waking to the place where I don't have to choose between being mortal and divine. It's a place where I don't have to know it all, and I can just be—a place of innocence. The naming of Eden, coming from the mouth of an innocent child, is perfect. There are so many connections. It's so whole that I can't even see all the way around it. It just keeps coming together."

We turn south beginning our descent toward home, following the geese. The path diverges. Bearing right would lead us to my old home, the Brown House. But I don't live there anymore; my DNA has changed its tune. Today we go left, by the old abandoned sugarhouse, across the small stream on wooden planks. We circle back to the path on which we started our journey.

"So how did this all come together? I mean, you must have been getting sick for a while, even before you remembered your birth in the ZB session because that was just a few months ago, right? And the miscarriage was a year ago," Kayla says.

"Yes. For my whole life, up until now, I was operating with the frequency given to me by my physical ancestors, passed along through DNA from generation to generation. It's as if my *unique* soul vibration didn't jell with my matter until now, so I've been getting along with what I've inherited. The timing makes sense to me astrologically and developmentally.

"Around the ages of thirty-eight to forty-two is a significant time. We have a potent opportunity to come in to the true expression of who we really are. It is the end of the first half of our lives and the beginning of the second half. I see it as a horizontal figure eight—the infinity symbol. At this time, where we are now, approaching age forty, we have moved along the left-hand circuit growing up, going to school, establishing careers, having children, and all that. Now we are back in the middle, at the crossroads of the figure eight. It is a natural time of rebirth. We either take what we have become and move on to a new expression of life, or we rehash and over manage the circumstances of our old lives. The former seems to lead to grace whereas the later leads to disintegration. For me, it's time to let go of the inherited energy of loss and futility and allow the clearer, stronger energy field of my soul, that is, my divinity, to integrate into my body. It's conscious evolution, Kayla!"

"It *is* conscious evolution, Shell," she says quickly. She is right there with me on the leading edge of my self-understanding. "And there's still a piece about the miscarriage I need to clarify. I can feel how essential it is, but I can't quite get there myself yet. Can you say anymore about that?"

"Well, the pregnancy was the unexpected answer to my prayers. What I wanted was the palpable sensation of the divine in my body. The goddess said, "I have just the thing to show her who she really is." In so many spiritual teachings there is the theme of coming home, and the idea that one comes home to her place with God. It is also usually the case that this homecoming requires a journey of some kind. I needed to experience all of the separation assumed at my core in order to see and feel my unity with the divine. I didn't need a pregnancy or another child to get it because I already had it. But, I didn't *believe* in it.

"The miscarriage was a great earthquake of grief. It cracked my veneer of perfection and my shell of righteousness. The crack went all the way to bone, into the very cellular matrix of my bones, and into my DNA. It went all the way to the core of who I am. It reopened all the fault lines within me that I had held glued together for a lifetime in fear of grief and sorrow and loneliness. Once opened, there was no gluing those faults back together. There was trying to glue it back, but awareness had snuck in between the surfaces. Awareness doesn't stick like glue. It's more like water. Awareness moves things. Even when I *pulled myself back together* some days after the miscarriage and returned to caring for my family and my patients, I was standing on shaky ground, slippery ground substance, shifting connective tissue.

"With all the aftershocks still reverberating in my bones, I asked for a big ZB session. I guess I knew somewhere in my heart that I wanted to break open. I wanted to see. I wanted to stretch and dance outside of the persona that I had nicely constructed for the past forty years. Re-experiencing my birth enable me to see the content inside my fault lines. It was all right there in my cells. I could see all the way into my DNA. I could see my ancestors, and I could understand the poverty, the pain, and the futility. More cracks started resonating open. All my cells, all my DNA were affected. Opened. Unzipped. Unwound.   I was suspended unzipped. I don't mean to say all of my DNA was physically separated, but it's more like my DNA was immobilized in a phase. Part of me was responding to the grief that has been exposed by climbing up above it, using all of my energy to tread water on the surface. Another part of me was underneath the surface, exploring the fissures. The belief that my soul was separate from my body was amplified.   It was time to sink or swim—time to surrender to my soul.   My soul was saying, "Die persona. Die stiff, immobilized, make-believe person. Die to me. Die to your soul!'"

Kayla stops in her tracks and turns to me. Her face is contorted by deep concentration and apprehension. "Okay, so wait. Why would your soul want you to die?"

"I must die to my soul. That is the journey. It

doesn't mean my physical body has to die. If I surrender to my soul, come back down into my body, into my bones, then *that* is the death, and I don't have to physically destroy myself. It's becoming clearer as we talk. It's a symbolic death. It's a homeopathic death."

We have come full circle and are standing, once again, on the sturdy wooden bridge behind the farmhouse. Kayla takes my hands in hers, forming a bridge of truth between us. She looks steadily and joyfully into my eyes, boring a hole into my cerebral cortex.

"You are creating your myth, Shell. You are really doing it. You are living your own myth."

My eyes smile deep into hers. "It's pretty cool." I laugh. "To watch it unfold and to receive it."

"Very cool. Very courageous."

We emerge from the wooded trail and head for the house.

"Oh! And of course right when all this is changing, right when I am leaving home so that I can come home, we actually sell our house and move into this great place while we build our new house, which is built from our dreams and intentions. Our evolved house. I'm building a new house as I'm building a new body. Isn't that perfect? It's all just so wild!"

"It *is* wild," she agrees.

The Apple and the Tree

The geese are calling out to us. The world is alive. It wants to inform us, but we are often focused on the form, the label, the diagnosis, and not on the information within the form. If we are present to hear the geese, look for the rainbows, can feel our bones and cells and DNA, then we are meeting the world. In this meeting, there is an exchange of awareness. We see the world and the world sees us. The geese have an offering. They say, "Yes! Your DNA changes." The Middle Meadow has a purpose. If I stopped and waited there until I got what I thought I wanted, I would have missed the geese. The world keeps moving. Our reference point is the point of profound stillness that comes with the awareness that we are one with the whole of the world.

Would we do better to stop trying to grasp and manipulate an external life? Maybe there is no use in trying to figure it out. Maybe there is no getting it right. It's as if we've come to the dance, but we've been sitting on the sidelines too long discussing the dance steps. Meanwhile, the band plays on, and the only ones who are having any fun are those who are dancing, those who are moving to their own rhythm, and those who say, "yes!"

How do we become so stiff and so focused on the external? We learn to be that way by identifying ourselves through the outer world. Early on, babies point and name. School children memorize mathematical facts and historical dates. We are taught to give up our imagination to the "reality" of life. The hard-and-fast, predetermined reality of someone else's life. Our eyes stiffen and lock, and our perception of the world changes. Yet we are still the world and are still moving beneath the illusion of determinism. Friction is created when the experiences of our lives scrape up against the fixed constructs we have come to believe. We create a struggle when we try to grasp the apple of knowledge and pluck it from the tree. We feel the apple in our hands and we "know" what it is. We also know we are narrowing our perspective to name it a small and solitary thing. It was so much more when it was still attached to the tree. How can we return to innocence when the apple is separate from the living, growing tree? We can tell our stories and dance our dance. We can learn to trust the sensory apparatus inherent in our bodies. We must regain the eyesight of a child, release the restrictions, and soften the constructs of our minds.

We can learn to hold both the structure of our lives and the energy of our lives simultaneously. When we bring awareness to both, the separation between spirit and matter disappears. Innocence and knowledge dance like Fred and Ginger. We are left to delight in the mesmerizing relationship of the whole. It is a very different way of being than sitting in the vacuum between the apple and the tree, or the chair and the dance floor.

What We Look For

Some weeks after the ZB session at Angel's Rest, I realized I was not thinking of myself as sick anymore. I was no longer unzipped. Threads of golden realizations, knitted together through the ZB session, pulled my DNA strands back around each other. Unity replaced separation as the signature of my cells. Now when people whispered with their genuine concern, "How are you doing?" I would say, "Good. That autoimmune thing is healed, and I feel great." Some smiled and probably wondered what I was talking about. Friends and family with health care backgrounds sort of looked at me sideways with doubt and questioning in their gaze. I explained that I had reprogrammed my DNA; I was no longer expressing the autoimmune tendency.

I don't think it is a widely held belief among scientists that we can consciously control gene expression. We have learned that we inherit genes from the chromosomes in our parents' cells. It is common knowledge that some genes predispose a person to certain conditions or diseases. Further, some genes are not expressed (turned on) until later in life. With autoimmune conditions, genes commonly begin to express in the fourth and fifth decade, and are most common in women. Why then? Why women? In my years of studying the human body, I have heard no explanation for why or how genes suddenly wake up and start wreaking havoc. I have only my own experience, and a solid appreciation for what I have learned about the human body from previous scientific investigation.

More recent research in the field of cell biology indicates there is a vibrational component to cell physiology along with the more mechanical models recognized in the past. It is now known that cells respond to our daily experiences, our emotions, thoughts, and beliefs. Cellular activity can be explored and partially explained through the mechanical and chemical models *and* there is new evidence suggesting that receptors on the surface of cells actually help mediate cellular resonance by changing their *vibrational* state.

The journey into my cells informs me we should be looking at cell biology more closely as a function of vibration or energy. As discussed earlier through the idea of cellular resonance, information can be passed through mechanical as well as through energetic forces. Quantum physicists tell us the universe is made up of tiny packets of light called quanta. All that we know, feel, see, and hear is made up of these quantum particles moving through space. The nature or reality of what we perceive is dependent upon the rate of vibration or the energy of these particles. In other words, our reality, our very physical reality, is based on the movement of light, the frequency of light, and largely on the amount of space between quanta of light. How we see the world around us is directly related to how much of this quantum nature we shine our awareness on. What we perceive depends on what we are looking for.

Our perception is more subjective than we realize on a daily basis. There is an Indian story about knowing an elephant. Several people are blindfolded and stand near an elephant. They are asked to describe what is in front of them. The first person, standing near a leg reaches out and feels the large, cylindrical, solid object and declares, "It's a column." The second, standing at the tail, says, "No, it's a rope." The third person, standing at the elephant's side proclaims that it is a wall. The fourth, near the trunk says, "It's a hose." When we step back and look at the bigger picture, we can see how easy it is to be mistaken. The elephant is none of those things. But what if we are *still* standing too close? If we step back even farther, or step deeper into our own experience, and look into her gentle knowing eyes, we may see she is more than a thing—more than a beast of burden, more than a wild animal, and more than a circus trickster. She is a being, a spirit, a soul. She is a vibration, an energy. She may offer us more than our initial cursory perception of her. She may offer us her experience. She may be sad or fierce and proud. Is she wise and elegant? When we step back from knowing, when we open ourselves to experience in the moment, we are informed with the kaleidoscope of vibration within our imaginations. Stories develop and unfold. The world comes alive. We wake up to a more liquid perception of life. The spirit of the world is right there waiting for a crack in the façade of our all-knowing human identities, offering a world of magic, connection, and synchronicity in which geese call out their encouragement and cats send messages from the afterlife, where lakes are alive, and rocks bear witness.

And what of ourselves? What can we experience of

ourselves? What can our bodies teach us about who we are? Can we feel ourselves in deeper ways? Can we embrace our own hearts? Can we clear our heads, soften our eyes, step back from who we think we are and feel beneath our beliefs to the raw and immediate nature of life? All matter is also energy. We have endeavored to keep matter and energy apart for decades after our beloved Albert Einstein told us that they are one— $E=mc2$. It has taken us close to a century to shift our perception enough to begin to consider life from this new perspective. We are energy. Life is vibration. The world is alive and interactive, responsive and malleable.

The Law of Similars

Winter of 2000 came and went in a frozen blur. The flowers began their annual push toward the light. Robins bobbed for worms once again. As the skeleton of the landscape faded behind new green leaves, the skeleton of our new home was emerging. Excavators dug into the clay of the earth as my awareness sunk deeper into the clay of my body. So many changes, so much new theory, a new way of seeing, and a new home, and yet something wasn't quite complete. I felt well but slightly tentative still.

A friend had given me the novel *The Law of Similars* by Chris Bojalian.[14] It is the story of a man's introduction to the world of homeopathy. Welcoming the distraction from the more heady material of science and spirit in which I am usually engulfed, I devoured the book in a couple of days and received a serendipitous suggestion. Oh, homeopathy. I don't know why I never really considered whether homeopathy could help me heal. I was familiar with homeopathic medicine from raising my children naturally, without drugs. We used over-the-counter homeopathic remedies for aches, colds, fevers, etc. I consulted a classical homeopath with good results when Beau began to suffer from ear infections as an infant.

Homeopathy is a philosophy of health and a formal system of medicine following principles developed by Samuel Hahnemann in the late eighteenth century. It is based on the principle of the law of similars, which is the theory that like cures like. In other words, a person will be cured by a proven remedy if the substance from which the remedy is made can produce the same specific symptoms (in a healthy person) as the person seeking the cure is expressing. The more closely the symptoms match, the more effective the remedy. As I understand it, the symptoms we express are our body's response to the *dis-ease* we are suffering. If we introduce a minute quantity of the substance which is a vibrational match to our symptoms (i.e., our body's natural corrective response) then that remedy will boost the body's innate healing response, offering a type of phase shift, and assist the body in getting to where it knows to go.

Inspired by a deeper experience with homeopathy through the main character of the book, I decided to seek the advice of the professional homeopath I had consulted years ago with Beau. Thus, the book itself was truly homeopathic—the story of a person's discovery of homeopathy caused a similar response in the reader.

Julian is a thin man. There is no extraneous stuff about him. He lives close to his skeleton, and he practices homeopathy in the same way. Eight years had passed since I last saw him, and I remembered a certain dryness to his manner. The day I walked into his office to explain the constitutional shift I felt was out there for me somewhere in the world of homeopathic remedies, I saw him differently. I had been immersed in the study and practice of hands-on energy work since our last meeting and so much had transformed already on this healing journey.

The whole world felt different now. *Julian is not dry. He's pleasant enough, but not overly friendly. He is interested in helping me. He is engaged. Ah, I know what it is. He is clear. No extra meat on the bone. He is core. No extraneous emotion or personal agenda comes to greet me. He meets me with his purpose. He is not particularly interested in befriending me. He does not concern himself with my approval. This is good. I don't need a buddy. I don't need him to like me or to believe my story. I need an expert homeopath. He shows up.*

The way I see it, the job of a classical homeopath is to listen deeply and ask clear questions, to excavate the bones of my constitution. The more I learned about healing, the more I aligned myself with healing techniques based on the client's personal experience. Julian listened to my symptoms, my dreams, my tastes, and my observations, and he searched his experience (and that of his laptop computer's) for a remedy having those same experiences as *proofs*. (A proof is a collection of data that has been carefully and repeatedly documented, listing the symptoms, experiences, and other phenomenon reported by healthy individuals given a dose of a particular remedy.)

I figured, the clearer the homeopath, the more accurately he could see me. He was concerned with precision. He searched for a remedy that matched my experience of myself and moved me further into a healthy expression of myself. Homeopathy fit with chiropractic, Zero Balancing, and the naturopathic approach I had been using. The basic assumption in all of these systems was that I was whole. I was well and right at my core. The therapeutic approach then, was to identify any interference to the free expression of my wholeness, to lift any physical, vibrational, emotional, mental, spiritual, nutritional, and metabolic interference that dampens my life force.

Fortunately or unfortunately, Julian had to sift through my whole long story to see the assembled puzzle. He listened patiently, occasionally nodding slightly or launching an interested eyebrow, as I reviewed the events of the past few years and how I felt at present.

"I feel that homeopathy has something to add. A phase shift into the wholeness of all of this," I said. *This poor guy,* I thought.

"Okay. Well..," he said slowly and evenly, "I think I have a good idea of what remedy I would recommend for you, but I want to think it over a little more. I'll send a remedy to you in the mail within the next few days."

Well, all right then.

Beavers and Balance

Two streams coursed through the property on which we were building our new home, and each had been damned by beavers. A family of beavers will build and inhabit a pond while clearing the view of saplings and an occasional full-grown tree. Gnawed off branched are inserted into the damn in a constant effort to maintain the depth of their pond. The stream, of course, has its own objective, which is to move. Beavers do not seem to mind their busy maintenance schedule. They build to eat and eat to build in a never-ending cycle of business. Rarely will I catch one lazily paddling around her pond, enjoying the fruits of her labor. And even then, although they are generally docile, they seem to become agitated if I catch them relaxing. They slap their paddle-shaped tails on the water to scare me away, as if they feel guilty for not working. Are beavers Irish?

There comes a time when enough trees have been taken that the edge of a balance point is reached. Beavers will take no more but will move upstream and start the building process all over again. They will be back next year or in several years or their offspring will. They offer a kind of reverse-habitat fulcrum—introducing the force of their teeth and their will, holding until a point of balance is brought to an edge, and making a clean, clear disconnect. I was supported by the lesson in sustainability from beavers: consume less than the amount that will upset balance. This was the medicine they offered to us as we built our home beside theirs.

The gift of having the Brown House on the market for four years was that we had lots of time to imagine our new house. Being drawn to the inherent rightness of all things natural, I researched how to build a house in harmony with the earth. I learned that some brave souls were building off-the-grid homes, which meant they were not connected to or dependent on large electric utilities for their power needs. Instead, they used renewable energy resources such as photovoltaic cells, wind turbines, geothermal heating, passive solar design, and solar hot water applications to create comfortable modern homes.

The idea of building an off-the-grid home appealed to me on many levels. At this point in the earth's history, when the supply of underground oil is declining, it seemed the only responsible thing to do was build with energy efficiency in mind. If we were off-the-grid, we would have to learn how to generate our own electricity and, more importantly, we would have to learn to use less electricity. We could have appliances like a dishwasher and a washing machine; we would just have to choose energy efficient ones. All our light bulbs would be compact fluorescent or low-voltage halogen. Yes, we would have to make lifestyle changes in order to live off-the-grid, and they were all changes I eagerly embraced. The simple choice to live off-the-grid would require us to live more consciously, and I like living consciously.

I assumed it would take a lot of convincing to get Dale to agree, so I did my homework. I read books on solar living and perused catalogues of energy efficient products. I filled out energy-use worksheets for our family's usage and consulted experts on the size of a photovoltaic system we would need to run our home/office. I calculated the cost of a free-standing renewable power source and compared it to what we would spend to get utility-generated power run to our somewhat remote meadow. When I approached Dale with a serious request to consider an alternative house, I had developed a solid vision. He was more receptive than I had anticipated. It would require more money up front but would pay for itself in ten to fifteen years. It would require some maintenance that he found acceptable. Dale did a little of his own research, could not find any contraindication, and agreed to build me my dream.

A similar course of events happened after I saw my first book on straw-bale construction. It was different, experimental, maybe even risky in New England, but technically, it made sense. We could build a strong wooden structure with lots of windows on the south side, envelope it with one-foot thick bales of straw, and plaster over them. We would have a passive solar house with an extremely high insulation value and plenty of stony mass to retain heat. It would be incredibly labor intensive and would offer walls with soft, organic curves, arches and nooks, deep-set windows, and cave-like rooms. Through our research, we found a straw-bale expert who lived less than thirty miles from us and had written a book on straw-bale construction for northern climates.

Dale and I agreed to be the next pair of beavers to inhabit the land. We would endeavor to build with respect for the earth and her resources. We would build a healthy house without toxic chemicals and fumes. We would build a simple structure that would be our workplaces as well as our home. We would build a home that was safe and nurturing and inspiring for our little beavers. We would build with balance.

Let It Come

The homeopathic remedy arrived in my post office box two days after consulting Julian. It was a fun piece of mail. The yellow padded mailing envelope looked at home and commonplace among the stack of business letters, bills, and Victoria's Secret catalogues. Without even being opened and consumed, it offered a unique vibration. I knew the information it contained was pure. It was not going to offer me underwear at a 20 percent discount or demand payment for telephone calls. Inside this little package was information in the form of pure vibration. Inside this envelope was the potential for more of myself. It was a phase shift transported right through the U.S. Postal Service.

At home, I peeled the gummy envelope open and inside found a smaller two-inch by three-inch white packet with instruction written on the front:

> Dissolve all pellets
>
> In one-quarter cup of water
>
> Take one teaspoon per day
>
> For three days

There was no explanation, no description, and no identification of what the remedy was. It was like receiving instructions for a secret mission. I had a fleeting vision of eating the envelope after I followed the instructions to destroy the evidence. Actually, I had expected this type of presentation, as a homeopath will often want the remedy to be experienced by a person without attachment to what it is supposed to do. ZB is much the same. It is offered as an experience, and it does not often serve the client to suggest how they will or should feel. Homeopathy works on the donkey level.

Lifting the fold on the small packet, I found fifteen to twenty tiny, round pellets that looked like round sugar granules. I dissolved them as instructed and faithfully took my teaspoon of energized water each day for the next three days. There was no immediate reaction to the remedy. Most of the major symptoms that had been disturbing me were no longer present, so I kept my inner awareness open for the more subtle whispers of change.

There is a timing and rhythm to the music of life, and we can enjoy it when we stay in our center and let it come to us. I would just wait for the wave of the remedy to come to me. In the meantime, the current song of life continued. We were rockin' and rollin.' The house was being prepared for the straw bale raising day when volunteers would join hands in wrapping the frame with insulating bales of straw. Urgency was the underlying tone and tempo. Summer was flowing on, and we would need to get the bales up and the plaster on before the cold weather moved in. It was a busy time. There was never any question of what to do with my time in those days. If I wasn't eating, sleeping, or tending to the needs of the boys, I was at the land building, building, and building. Like the beavers, there was so much work to do that at a certain point I just gave up on the idea of ever finishing. Not that I thought we wouldn't finish, but I just had to start building for the sake of building and let go of the outcome. It was too exhausting trying to reach for the end all the time.

Breath of Love

It was Saturday morning, about a week after taking my homeopathic remedy, and I awoke in the farmhouse feeling light. The smell of freshly brewing coffee and the song of boyish laughter seeped into the room. Lying in bed on my back, I was flooded with gratitude for all the lightness and all the rightness in my life.

We are building our house. We will be living on this property that is so beautiful and so abundant. Dale and me—two kids from the shorter side of middle class America...who would have thought? And then, after a pause to take it all in...*well there's plenty of work to do today, so up you go.*

I rolled onto my side and sat up. The gratitude followed and liquid light poured into my belly like cold beer into a frosty mug. I was being filled up. I sat on the bed for a minute, with my feet on the floor, just noticing how happy I was. Something was different. As I slowly stood up, what I can only describe as a rush of golden love flowed into the top of my head and down through my body to me feet. My heart opened in a new way and allowed blood to flow more freely. In that moment I was acutely aware of the connections between the physiology and the mythology of my heart. I felt the blood pulsing everywhere in my body with each heartbeat. I felt love being pumped into my flesh with each pulse. I was being breathed into like Adam or Eve. I was a vessel of divine love. I was being chosen, again.

The room became still and silent. I lost all sense of

time and space. I stood motionless receiving a strange and sublime combination of the softening of my heart tissue and the sharpening of my hearts ability to feel. The earth's gravitational field pulled waves of warmth down into my feet, and the heavenly bodies sucked it back up. Together they danced a beautiful figure eight of fluid love that became one in my heart.

So humble, I whispered through quivering lips as my palms met in front of my heart. *I am so humbled.* "Thank you, thank you," I said aloud into my hands.

Humble feels like happy where I am. Not striving or searching but receiving the gifts of the world and feeling innately satisfied. Humble feels grounded and open and safe, innocent, and childlike. It feels like being rewarded for believing in my own safety and my own divinity.

This is my remedy. It has opened me to unity in a sensory way. I can physically feel more of my heart. More dimensions of my heart's function.

Raising Bales

There is a beginning, middle, and an end to each Zero Balancing fulcrum. The practitioner introduces a force around which the body can reorient, holds a point of stillness for seven to ten seconds or the approximate time it takes to count "hold it, hold it, hold it," and then makes a clean, clear, disconnect. Our farmhouse was a two-year point of relative stillness. It was stillness in the sense that we stayed there in temporary suspension while we did the work to come into our new and more authentic home. Near the end of the construction process people would ask, "Are you in your new house yet?"

"Not quite."

"Almost."

"Soon."

It sounded like the hold it, hold it, hold it of a ZB fulcrum. I would be working in my office or shopping in the supermarket or watching a soccer game, and while it may have looked like nothing significant was happening to me, there was an intense metabolic churning within as the structure and energy of my body reorganized simultaneously with the organization of the structure and energy of my new home. It was a working state.

It was a time of constant focusing and refocusing of attention. Get the boys fed and off to school. See patients all day. Feed the kids dinner. Get homework done, sports schedules coordinated, birthday parties attended, new shoes obtained, volunteer work done, and *then* get to the land.

Call Diana to dowse the well location. Get quotes on the well. Bless the well. When are the cement contractors coming to pour the foundation? Be at the house when the cement is still wet. Set crystals and draw runes in the four directions in the still malleable stone. Pray and bless the foundation. Organize contractors. Choose, choose, choose—with care. What color for the metal roof, the crown of our home? Ah! They have indigo—perfect! Do I dare have an indigo roof? Green is okay. It would blend in with the surroundings, after all integration with the natural world is a central principle on which this house is built. But that doesn't feel right. It's safe but not right. I'm going with my heart on this one. Indigo. Okay, that's settled. The framing is done, and the wooden structure is beautiful standing in a green spring meadow. When to have the straw delivered? How to keep it dry? Organize the straw-bale raising day. Ask for help (gulp!). Ask for help again. Ask for help again. Okay, that's not so hard now.

The skeleton of the house was assembled. A striking indigo metal roof became one more peak in the twilight majesty of the Green Mountains. Five hundred and twenty bales of wheat straw, grown in northern Vermont arrived in an eighteen wheeler and were stacked inside the frame to keep dry. The next step was the bale raising, which is the process of enveloping the bones of our home with straw bales. Efficiency was critical now. Keeping the bales dry was of paramount importance. We would need to put them in place and prepare to plaster over them before the weather turned too wet or too cold. We planned to have a bale-raising weekend. Friends and family were notified months earlier that at some point they would be invited to get their hands in the building process. Most were eager to help, and some were excited to learn an innovative building technique. Only a few people treated us as if we were trying to get free help, which hurt temporarily. But when you are building a house, there is just too much to do to allow time spent worrying about yesterday. So any misunderstanding and anything less than positive was given a gracious nod and not a backward glance.

One cannot impose a date on the organic becoming of a house—at least not this one. It would let us know when it was ready to receive its flesh, its walls, and its containment. Our straw-bale consultant, Paul, showed us how to stack and secure the bales to the frame. When the timing was right we would teach any willing body how to follow suit.

When the house was ready, Labor Day weekend arrived without the clutter of clouds, rain, high winds, or lightening. Mother Earth was there to help along with the friends and family that poured into the driveway. With each face I greeted that morning, the warmth of humility burrowed deeper into my grateful heart. Brothers, sisters, nieces and nephews, parents, friends, friends, and more friends, friends of friends, children of friends, patients, colleagues, Zero Balancers, the owner of the building supply store, a yoga teacher, and women from council. Some came to get their hands in the straw, and some came to feed us. Some came to play in the field. I was so happy to receive this blessing of human hands and human hearts; I felt like a queen at a parade all day, as I greeted, smiled, and acknowledged. This new ability to feel so humble and to receive so much was breaking my heart open and love was pouring from all directions into the walls of my new home.

Those who arrived early in the morning were asked to begin with intention. We gathered in a circle and held hands. I thanked everyone for their presence and told them that we were building a house with positive energy. We explained that we had asked each of them if they would like to help because we felt their hands and hearts could add value to our home. There was only one basic rule: work with happiness, and if you are not having fun, take a break.

"No cursing into the walls of my house!" I admonished with a smile.

We spent many, many hours considering the energy of this structure. The floor plan was laid out in a way that was efficient for the way our family moved. Materials were chosen not only for their function but for their form, feel, color, texture, scent (or lack thereof), and beauty. We had many, many meetings with our friend and architect, Joseph, as we felt our way through our home and described our dance, so he could assist us in matching the structure of the walls, windows, roof, and deck, to our dreams and visions.

As the bale raising day progressed, I greeted and steered volunteers toward groups of people already at work. Receiving, receiving, and receiving the gift of human support, and trusting human hands. I was coming down into myself and out of the clouds to feel love come to me; I was falling into myself, falling in love with life, and feeling gratitude and humility snuggled securely in my bones. When I stacked and cinched and strapped the straw into the walls that day, I put deep peace and acceptance, gratitude, humility, and a whole lot of smiles into the walls of my house.

Julie was clear that her work was not heaving bales of hay. "That's just not my kind of thing," she said. "But, I'll organize the food. I'm good at organizing and good at food!"

By lunchtime there were three canopies set up over tables laden with more food than the whole crew could eat. There were platters of fruits and vegetables, salads of all kinds, breads, crackers and cheese, tasty sweets, and coolers full of beverages. Flowers adorned tables, and Marietta came wearing her summer bonnet. It looked more like a lawn party than a construction site. The feast added the energy of grace, beauty, and abundance to the physical, sweaty, itchy and rewarding work of stacking and securing bales of straw on a hot summer day.

The Medicine of One

Six weeks after taking the homeopathic remedy, I returned to Julian's office for a follow-up.

"So, how are you doing?" he asked.

"Good," I said cheerfully. "You know, I was already feeling good when I took the remedy, so mostly what I was aware of was this feeling of being humble."

"Humble?" Julian stated and asked simultaneously, launching a particularly interested eyebrow.

"Yeah, like this pouring of God's attention into my life. It's a grounded feeling. It's not that I wasn't humble, but now that I feel this way, I can tell that I was operating in something other than this vibration for a long time. It feels like I must have been striving a lot before, and now I'm just here, and it's all coming to me."

"Huh. Anything else?"

"Well, yes, I haven't been worried about money. I just seem to notice financial concerns arising, and then I move on, trusting that all will be provided. Somehow that is a lot easier now."

"Hmmmm."

Julian's frequent "hmmms" and "ah-huhs" were often followed by long periods of silence—the kind of silence that typically makes people squirm. The kind of silence that can feel like it needs to be filled. The kind of silence that is often socially awkward when it strikes distance between two people who are trying to relate. But I wasn't uncomfortable with his silence. It was familiar to me. It is the silence of mental churning, the silence of the type of decision making that I was used to in my own practice. It was Julian sifting and sorting both the information I was offering and the knowledge that he had collected through his professional experience. Today, Julian's "hmmm" was followed by the faintest smile. *He knows he has the right remedy!*

"So," he said slowly, "the remedy I gave you was hydrogen."

"Hydrogen? I didn't know they made remedies from hydrogen!"

"Yes, it's fairly new work. Some contemporary homeopaths have done provings on the whole periodic table. It's quite fascinating."

"Hydrogen. It seems so simple. So basic."

"Yup. Its number one in the periodic table," he said, holding up a single index finger.

"Oh! The unity thing! That's cool!"

"It's interesting," he continued, "I thought hydrogen was the remedy for you when we met, but I wanted to check further. I didn't know it at the time, but I found that one of the characteristics of a hydrogen person is a fear of poverty. So that sounded like a good match."

"Huh!" was all I could manage.

"The fact that you feel humble is also very interesting to me. Another trait of hydrogen was described as spiritual haughtiness. Now, I wouldn't have thought you spiritually haughty from our interactions, but what you are saying about this overall feeling of humility suggests that perhaps you are moving away from spiritual striving."

"Yeah, I feel like it's all been given to me. I don't have to reach up into the sky for God anymore. I have *received* a connection with the divine.

"Good," he said cheerfully. "Anything else?"

I laughed, and we both knew there was no way that I could ask for more.

"No. I can feel that I got what I came here for and that the remedy will keep revealing itself to me."

He nodded.

"So, just the one dose? Do I have to take a maintenance dose or is that it?"

"I don't think I would suggest another dose right now. Like you said, let's give this one some time. Maybe check in with me in six weeks or so, and we'll see how it's going."

The phase shift had occurred. I did not need to support myself with a remedy. It was a shift in my constitution, and it was well received and integrated. It was *in* me now. It *was* me now.

Parallel

Summer moved steadily toward autumn as we surrendered to the never-ending task of building our home. Close to half of the bales were in place after the bale raising weekend. Dale worked daily, continuing to stack bale on top of bale. In the evenings, after working on bodies all day, I would labor with him.

Although the bales were packed very tightly and cinched together with strapping, there were occasional little spaces between that needed to be stuffed with loose straw. There was always at least one unbound bale cracked open on the floor from which to pull loose straw. Paul showed us how to make straw knots. Take a handful of loose straw as if grasping enough uncooked spaghetti for one serving and bend it as if breaking the pasta in half. Of course, straw is flexible, so it doesn't break, it folds. Next, twist it and fold it back on itself another time. The result is a knot of straw that looks like a casually disheveled chignon. The twisted straw knots are stuffed into any spaces between the bales. Usually thoughts are stuffed in there with them. I always tried to bring myself to peace when building the walls of my house. Stuffing the walls was like putting a child to bed. One knot was a bedtime story, the next was tucking him in, and the next was a kiss goodnight. There is always more opportunity to love.

As I stuffed straw into walls, I continued to stuff nutrients into my once-depleted body. I was unified with my body; I could no longer deny it. With each egg, each glass of water, each salad, and each vitamin capsule, I was adding love to this newly built body, this new me.   Cold air descended on Vermont, and we prepared to wrap the exposed flesh of our home in a blanket of new skin.   Paul assembled a hopper-style sprayer with which to spray the first coat of plaster right into the straw.   He made two huge wooden boxes and mixed the plaster recipe in them.   The first coat is a clay plaster: ground clay, sand, lime, chopped straw, and water.   Cells, collagen, DNA, plasma—it's all the same thing.

Plastering

Applying the first coat of plaster was a painfully slow process. Paul and his crew were great people to work with, but their work ethic was less influenced by economics other than ours. Every grain of sand slipping through the slender neck of the hourglass was a penny, a nickel, or a dollar. I wanted to pinch the waist of the hourglass to stop the erosion of our financial resources. Simultaneously, I wanted to speed up time and find myself at the end of the process.

Studying Zero Balancing, I had learned that when two opposite ideas, emotions, or beliefs are encountered simultaneously, it is impossible for our conscious mind to hold them both as true. The mind will go into an altered state of awareness. We go to a third place, a clean slate, which is informed by both of the beliefs that led us there but is limited by neither. I couldn't stop time, and I couldn't make it go faster. Trying to hold both desires brought me to a third place—surrender.

The house had its own becoming. We called it into being with our dreams and hopes and prayers. We consulted the animal world, the plant world, and the mineral world. We asked the earth where to drill the well and where to site the house. We invoked the seven directions, welcomed our ancestors, and invited angels and benevolent spirits. We honored the sun and the moon. We asked for the blessing of God, the goddess, Jesus, Hanuman, Ganesh, Sai Baba, Mother Mary, Artemis, and all the other guys and gaias we knew might well bestow blessings. Many expert midwives were in attendance, so all we could do was trust the natural birth process and go with the flow.

After four weeks, we did have our first coat of "mud" sprayed, toweled, and scratched (the process of raking the wet plaster to raise ridges on which the next coat could adhere). Both the interior and exterior walls were lumpy, bumpy, and brown, with pink splotches here and there above windows and over arches, where we added ground bricks to the mud to increase stiffness. That was all we could do on the exterior for the year; the frost was on the pumpkins, and it was too cold to apply the finish coat. We went through that first winter with a house that looked like it was made out of corrugated cardboard and patched with pink bubblegum. It was as if the house was born with its ancient soul-skin, a wrinkly newborn baby, a continuum of wisdom and innocence. Thank the goddess and Julian for that homeopathic dose of humility.

During the winter months, we spent long hours troweling the interior walls with a finish coat of lime plaster—what a mess! We mixed sand, lime, and water in wheelbarrows with a hoe and a hose, inside the house. I had unending opportunities to be astonished at the calm in my heart, my perseverance and patience, and the ability to choose not to be stressed. My work in the healing arts, integrating body, mind, and spirit through chiropractic and Zero Balancing was in precise alignment with my inner growth. The more I served to create ease, balance, and harmony in others, the more grace I experienced myself. I found my groove, and over time that groove deepened and resonated more with every fiber of my being. It was getting easier and easier to find comfort in almost any challenge.

In the process of plastering, I began to really feel the vibration of our new house. The work became less about finishing a project and more about service. It became devotional work like polishing the back of the Buddha. When I started plastering, it was just the job that needed to be done at the time, but I soon began to experience plastering as a conversation with structure, much like working on a body. I felt as though I was in service to the spirit of the house. As I assisted in creating form, I was informed by the interface of my body and the walls. I could hear thoughts and ideas that didn't seem to be solely mine. As I lifted a scoop of plaster onto my trowel and drew it upward from the base of a wall, I felt uplifted, too. It was like helping a child up a step. *Take my hand. Up you go. There you are.* Sometimes, when I was very weary or when I began to worry, the walls would comfort me. *It's all right. You are on track. Keep going. Be patient. Remember magic.* Slowly, as I listened to the walls coming to life, the realization crystallized: there is a return for intention. I was in touch with the energy of the house! Prayers, blessings, and invocations were the tools of building a structure which holds intention. Our love, respect, and care were actually held in the hardened plaster of the walls. And the walls could give back. The house was awake and held us in the arms of our own intentions.

One wall a day. One room a week. We plastered

for over two months. Lime plaster is dusty when dry, caustic when wet, and heavy in either state. The upside to aching muscles, burning fingers, and desiccated skin was that the walls were literally plastered with love, with hope, and with prayers. Each wall had thoughts, patience, care, and dreams pressed into it. The walls were plastered with music and were sung into being. They were touched and formed with human awareness, with consciousness. Despite my admonitions, a few curses probably found their way in there, too. Balance, you know. Real life. The shadow and the light. The moon and the sun. Yin and Yang. Ben and Jerry.

The day I plastered the Zero Balancing room in my office, I was listening to a recording of Krishna Das singing spiritual chants. As I sang along, I thought lovingly of Kayla, my dear friend who had moved to her homeland, an island in Puget Sound. She had introduced me to this Sanskrit chanting in yoga class. She played Baba Hanuman while we were in a long restorative pose. I had never heard anything so beautiful! Krishna Das's voice went right to my heart and broke it open. Now, plastering and chanting, the tears flowed down my cheeks, onto my trowel, and were firmly pressed into the limestone. They were tears of praise and joy, evoked by this deep rich voice calling out the God in my bones. There were tears of gratitude for the gift of a friend like Kayla who completely understood the tenderness in my heart. The gelatin of my heart was melted into a river of love that rippled through my arms and into the flat metal blade as it massaged the cavern of my sacred workplace into being.

It is one of the smoothest walls in the house.

Kayla lived in the valley for years and still owned her house in Vermont; she returned to visit for a few weeks over the winter holidays. We were eager to spend some time catching up with each other. I was continuously working on the house, so we planned a work date.

She arrived looking down-to-earth chic in her orange parachute pants, pink and orange skin-tight polyester T-shirt, with just the right curve at the neckline, and her shoulder-length blond hair a perfect mess. We fell into the curves of each other's bodies, the full-bodied feminine greeting that had become our ritual. After approving of new hairstyles and generally agreeing that we both looked great, we were ready to get down to work. We scavenged a pair of old work boots from the shoe closet and a coverall from Dale's shop. I demonstrated the ins and outs of lime plastering, and we decided to start working on the archway leading from the foyer into my office. As we began to plaster, Kayla admired the form of the arch, and we spoke of how it functioned as a portal between the external world and the womblike space of my office. If felt so right to be honoring the form and function of this particular structure as we were solidifying it's presence on earth. We also talked of families, relationships, and world service. We shared the details of each other's latest discoveries about life, spirit, and healing.

Kayla and I often explored animal medicine while hiking together. Observing our interaction with each other, we realized that human animals have their own unique medicine. For her fortieth birthday, I made an animal card out of one of the blank cards in the medicine card deck. I glued a picture of the two of us within the empty circle and wrote the word for the quality of human medicine as we had come to experience it: reflection. I presented it to her with a pair of earrings formed by interlocking a silver hoop and a gold hoop, signifying our connected journeys through the portals of our lives. Kayla and I were as different as silver and gold; she was vivacious, bold, and gregarious while I was grounded, quiet, and self-contained. We resonated in such a way that we reflected each other's essence. I could see how she saw me and loved myself more for the reflection. She would say the same.

As we continued to sculpt the archway, Kayla became more and more enchanted with the house. She was beginning to have her own conversation with the walls and was truly thrilled to be putting herself into the form.

"Will you name the house?" she asked.

"I don't know," I said. "I've been thinking about that. I've always felt that naming a house was presumptuous or pompous or something. But, I have to say, it seems to want a name. It's as if a name is being called forth—like it's already there, but I can't quite hear it. It's not a name based on the features of the land like Misty Meadows or Green Acres. It's something that feels a little mysterious like another world. Something like Avalon, but that's not it."

She turned to me, her trowel suspended in midstroke. "It's Eden."

The room became immediately silent and completely still. "Oh, My, God."

Eureka

I hate to admit it, but I gave up the fight on gun control a few years ago. The boys grew up on Bambi and Fantasia, but somehow, somewhere they learned how much boys need guns. Most mothers of young boys know what I'm talking about. I'll never forget the look of sheer delight on Justin's face the first time he bit his peanut butter toast into the shape of a gun. That's when I knew it was genetic. In the woods, there are sticks in the shape of every conceivable type of gun: pistols, rifles, and bazookas. In the toy aisle of the local variety store, they ran to the guns.

"Oh, I want that!" they sang in harmony.

At first it was easy. "No guns. Nope. Because we don't do guns. We don't have guns in our house. We are a gun-free family. Guns are violent. No. You know I don't like guns. That's it. No guns."

They just knew it as a rule. They never completely accepted it, but they couldn't overrule me at that time. They hadn't learn to reason with me and they still believed that I was the authority in their lives. By the time Justin was thirteen, most of his friends had either BB guns or paintball guns.

"C'mon, Mom. I'm old enough. I can be responsible. I'll show you. It's not violence. It's target practice. I won't shoot anything living, just the target," he said.

For another year it was still no, no, no, no and no, until one afternoon when Dale stopped by a nightclub in which he was installing a lighting system with the boys in tow. Wandering around the darkened room, while their father talked business they found an old BB gun behind a stack of bar stools.

"You want it?" the club owner asked.

Dale, also possessing the Y chromosome, simply refused to intervene. As they got older, they asked to go to movies that their friends were seeing. Most of them featured futuristic, technologically enhanced, bad guys with assault weapons. This led to another version of the same conversation all over again.

"Is it a violent movie?"

"Kinda."

"Why do all the movies you want to see have shooting and guns? I don't like violent movies."

This is where they learned to reason with me. "It's just a movie, Mom. It's not real. They are just actors. The bad guys are robots, and they just shoot the robots, so they don't take over the world. It's about saving humans and stopping the bad guys."

"Why do they have to kill them? Why don't they just turn them into good guys somehow? If you always see violence you'll think that's the right response, but violence creates more violence. Violence isn't creative, and it's stupid."

"We know, Mom," they would say with feigned sympathy. "But, we know better. It's just a movie. So, can we go?"

✶✶✶✶✶✶✶✶✶✶✶✶✶✶✶✶✶✶✶✶✶✶✶✶

It was a lovely early summer evening, perfect for bloodshed and destruction, when the boys asked to go to a new movie where robots vie for world domination. After the obligatory question and answer period, complete with begging and pleading, I agreed to drive them the twenty minutes to the theater. I didn't want to make two round trips, so I grabbed an old biology textbook and my notebook. My minivan is quite comfortable, and it stays light until about nine o'clock at that time of year, so I decided to do some research.

The story of DNA unwinding came to me as a personal experience, a deep knowing, and I trusted that. However, I was also curious about how my experience would tie into mainstream scientific knowledge. I majored in biochemistry as an undergraduate student, and I retained rusty scraps of information and cobweb-covered images of DNA replication, RNA transfer, and gene expression. I had to go back to the books to see if the information there would corroborate my story.

When we arrived at the movie theater, the boys stashed their water bottles into cargo pant pockets, and dashed to the ticket window. I slid my seat back from the steering wheel, reclined it slightly, crossed my legs in the lotus position, and opened the old biology text *Matter, Energy, and Life* by Jeffrey Baker and Garland Allen[15] to the chapter titled Nucleic Acids.

I reviewed the function of the two nucleic acids DNA and RNA. DNA is basically thought of as information storage units located in chromosomes within cell nuclei. RNA has more various and mobile functions and can be found both inside and outside of the cell nucleus. RNA communicates with the more fixed DNA, transcribing the information within DNA into proteins, the molecules of action. The more I read, the more excited I became. It was like being led along in a mystery; I was anticipating the solution, the coherence of all the evidence, and that one last piece of information that made it all fit together. I read that for DNA to replicate, or for RNA to transcribe from DNA, the DNA double strand must unzip to expose the sequence of nitrogenous bases at its core. .

The separation of the DNA strands can also be brought about by decreasing the concentration of various ions or by increasing the temperature. I thought about the illness on my due date, when I had a high temperature for four days. I considered the changing ion concentration (pH) in my blood stream as it was saturated with salicylic acid. Continuing on, I read that experiments had been performed that suggested RNA has an influence on DNA under certain conditions, perhaps by altering the base sequence when it pairs up. So influences from outside of the nucleus can get to the DNA and change its expression. Mmm-hmmm.

Then my eyes fell across a beautiful line of text that told me the unwinding of the two complimentary strands of DNA is a result of the breaking of hydrogen bonds between base pairs. *Of course, hydrogen bonds. Hydrogen!*

I had not considered the physical role of hydrogen in the winding or unwinding of DNA. This delightful piece of biochemical information was the gem I didn't know I was looking for. Although my homeopathic remedy of hydrogen essentially did not contain any molecules of hydrogen, it did hold the vibration of hydrogen—the vibration responsible for bringing the two separate strands into the unifying molecule of all life. Spirit had carried me this far, and now science was along for the ride. I had often described myself as one who loved the juxtaposition of spirit and science. No wonder. They had been held together all this time in my DNA by hydrogen.

Everything I Always Wanted

I felt like a kid in a candy store. Actually, I felt like a young, small-town girl at a shopping mall with my wealthy and generous aunt. I grew up on hand-me-downs and hand-sewn jumpers, discount store specials and slightly irregulars. But in my early teens, my Aunt Juju began the tradition of taking my older sister, Leslie, and me to the Burlington Mall before Christmas each year to pick out our presents. In the early 1970s malls were not a place where young girls hung out.

Just walking into Filenes' was a culture shock. Our eyes lit up at the mazes of shiny chrome racks laden with the latest styles; our heartbeats synchronized with the sound of coat hangers clacking as seasoned shoppers rejected one garment after another in search of just the right thing.

"Pick out whatever you like," my aunt encouraged us. Leslie and I modestly searched the chrome jungle for cool clothes that weren't too expensive. "Never mind the price tags!" Juju would scold us as we passed on the clothing that was marked anything over the median range.

We chose bell bottoms and polyester paisley blouses with macramé belts. Corduroy jackets with furry trim around the collar and sleeve. We thought we had died and gone to heaven. Anything we wanted could be ours. Of course, we argued with her all night; we were brought up to be frugal.

"You like that one, honey?   Good, now pick out another outfit."

"No, Juju. This is good. This is all I need."

"Okay, we'll go to Jordan Marsh, then, and see what they have."

It wasn't so much that we got new clothes, and we were going to look really good when we went back to school, it was the feeling of endless possibility. It seemed like the whole universe was contained in that shopping mall, and we were free to take it.

Now, sitting in the movie theater's parking lot, I had that same feeling of endless possibilities. My heart began to race, and my face flushed with the exhilaration of truth. Everything I had experienced through the eyes of Eden was validated again. Not that I needed much external validation; I knew by now this healing story was the right one for me. Synchronicities, correlations, supportive data, and connections just kept tumbling in to place, and my heart laughingly went galloping along for the ride. What fun to hold innocence and experience as one and learn there is no need to choose between them; to wonder how life could be if we humans would endeavor to trust our own experiences and hone our awareness to simplicity, so that we could rest our weary minds and let our feelings move us forward. Wouldn't most people be more at peace if they didn't have to decide so much by weighing external facts and figures? Is it possible that our success is built right into our lives, and we've been so busy trying to figure out how to get it right, that we've missed the roadmap right there in our hearts?

I had struck gold finding hydrogen, the element of unity, as the glue in my DNA. I had to put my book down. So much energy was coursing through me; I was vibrating with discovery, with understanding, and with the ring of truth. It felt great, but grounding would be necessary if I wanted to continue studying for the next hour. I headed to the nearby convenience store and let my heart lead me around until I was face to face with the ice cream freezer. What was that? Yin and yang? Right and wrong? Oh, yeah—Ben and Jerry's! I paid for chocolate covered ice cream on a stick and returned to the parking lot. I was ready to take notes.

It was dusk when the boys came running out of the theater and jumped into the car.

"How was the movie?" I asked.

"Good!" said Justin. "Actually, Mom, I think you would like it even though it had violence. It really makes you think about being human, about right and wrong, and how humans can wreck the earth and destroy themselves because they're not really being aware, even though they think they are being the good guy. You know what I mean?"

"Because there's a bigger picture of life that they're not seeing?"

"Yeah!"

"Yeah, I know what you mean," I laughed.

Crossing Over

First we thought we'd be in the house by November, then it was Christmas, but January rolled past, and we were still on our hands and knees tiling the floors. "Beau's eighth birthday, February tenth—we'll be in our new house for Beau's birthday," I said. Beau and I did sleep at the new house on his birthday, but we had to fold a futon, comforter, and pillows into the back of the car and drag them up the stairs to his new room. The plumbing and heating systems were up and running, but there was nothing else in the house except tools, building materials, and construction dust. It was very exciting. It was very quiet. We were very happy.

By late March, the kitchen was finally complete. On a Thursday afternoon, as Dale was finishing up some odds and ends at the new house, I began the process of packing at the farmhouse. Julie had a few hours to spare that afternoon and volunteered to help pack. She's a Virgo and is good at packing and organizing. It seemed the kitchen was the place to start since it required the least explanation. I already gave away everything we didn't actually use in the kitchen, so there wasn't much to pack. We packed things into big cardboard boxes because we only had to load them into the back of my minivan and drive three miles to the new house. We emptied and cleaned the refrigerator and the cabinets, filling more boxes. Within a few hours, we had moved the contents of our kitchen to Eden. As the last box went into the van, I turned to Julie.

"I don't know how we are going to cook dinner without any pots or pans.... wait a minute! If the home is where the hearth is and if the only kitchen that we can operate in is the one in the new house, then...we've moved! Oh-my-God, Julie, you just did it again. You totally midwifed me over another threshold. You've moved me in one day!"

"I guess we have!" she agreed.

"I'm shocked. I had no idea. I just didn't realize that it could be so simple. I didn't know what we were doing...I had this idea of an arduous two weeks of sorting and packing and now we are there looking back from the other side. I mean, sure, there is lots of ferrying of stuff still to do, but our base of operations is now Eden. This is totally your magic, Julie. It's like all the huffing and puffing of moving through labor, and then we just slip to the other side, where we are different— we are mothers. That's how I feel right now. I feel so relieved."

"Congratulations!" she said with a big, kind, knowing smile.

We parted ways with laughter, and I drove the last few boxes of kitchenware to our new home. When I informed Dale that we now lived at the new house, we decided we should have something to sleep on. He took off in his truck, wrench in hand, to disassemble our bed. He returned an hour or so later with the bed, along with sheets, blankets, pillows, and towels. The boys still had the futon from Beau's birthday sleepover to share until we got Justin's bed moved. It was a perfect first night in Eden.

Back to the Garden

When I opened my eyes the next morning, a vibrant spring meadow welcomed my waking through the window beside my bed. No shades were drawn, and there were no curtains to keep out unwanted distractions. I wanted it all—the stars, the moon, the birdsong, the trees, the breeze, the dawning day, and the sunrise. I was more alive than ever. I swear I could feel the roll of the earth toward the sun. I was greeted by the spring call of a chickadee, which in the birding books is referred to as *fee-bee* but sounds to me more like a melodic *you-who*. Chickadees always seem to want my attention. *You-who. Wake-up. List-en. Spring-sprung.*

Of course the seasons change in Vermont like they do elsewhere because the earth waltzes around the sun in a yearly cycle. It is a graceful and steady dance. Still, there is a day each spring when everything seems to shift suddenly. Chilly winter winds are blown away by balmy spring breezes. The earth stirs from her winter nap and yawns. Her breath rises from the thawing ground with the sweet scent of virgin green. The heady, fertile, enticing aroma of freshly brewed mud hangs low in the air. Brooks and streams skip and chatter, celebrating the snowmelt. A mysterious happiness fills the hearts of children causing them to turn off televisions and go running outside, which, in turn, fills the hearts of parents everywhere with even more mysterious happiness.

I rose and walked naked out into the living room

and stood in front of the wall of glass that looks southward across the meadow. I was struck by the paradox that I was at once *alone* with nature and *all one* with nature. With that contradiction resonating in my chromosomes, the false paint of illusion was gently rubbed off, and there I was, restored, in the original masterpiece of the Garden of Eden, where somehow I knew I had always belonged. I was home. *This is so perfect. Spring has dawned on our first day in our new house. The world is opening her arms to us.*

So strong was the feeling of interaction with the world that I felt I was alive within an Alex Grey drawing, all energy lines and grids were turned on and palpable. And then I realized: *It's Easter weekend! Easter! The Christian celebration of the resurrection of Christ. When the spirit of Christ rose from his earthly form and filled the heavens. The honoring of the everlasting bridge between heaven and earth. The shedding of the old cloak and stepping into a new life. The archetypical time of coming home. And the spring equinox! The time when the days are as long as the nights. The hopeful return of green life to the fertile valley. Easter bunnies. Fertility. The fruits of the union of male and female. Sun and moon. Heaven and earth. Unity and duality. Eden. This is all so right.*

Once again the story came around to wholeness. All chapters led to here and now, this eternal place and time that is no place and no time. My whole life conspired to help me get here. I was waking to Eden, back to the garden. I thought I had been seeing the world clearly, and then the focus was adjusted once again. I could see that my birth, my childhood, my family, my education, my marriage, my children, my miscarriage, my illness, and my new house—everything was in perfect order to bring me to the awareness that Eden is not only a mythical place. Eden is a possibility of living in heaven and earth at the same time. It is open to all because it is a personal experience that only requires the innocence of spirit to open to what the world has to offer. It only requires descent from the mind, dissolution of the ego, and the willingness to surrender to our place in the order to the world. Like Mary Oliver's "Wild Geese," "you only have to let the soft animal of your body love what it loves."[16]

This world is my home. Eden is my home, my house, my land. Not mine by possession but the one I see, the one I choose, the one in which I exist. It is a new dimension, a lane change, an altered perception. Eden is a place where spirit speaks and listens. Eden is alive and responsive. It is the same planet I inhabited before I was reborn except now we have awakened each other. There are new possibilities and different rules of engagement. It is a new world right beside the old one. It is a place where animals talk and plants offer their assistance, where the sun shines brighter, and the trees are more alive. Eden is a place of innocence and a place of humility, and a place of equality and a place of acceptance. It is a place of unity, and it has been here all along, waiting for my return from the proverbial fall from grace. I don't have to be a fallen sinner. I am Eve. I know Adam. Our union was blessed by God with children. Sexuality is sacred. Fertility is a blessing. I am awake, and I am innocent. I am not wrong! I am not broken! I am whole. I have been given consciousness, so that I can make my way back to the wholeness, the beauty, and the blessing of another beautiful day on earth.

Hello, grace. I'm back. I am waking to Eden; my eyes are open, and it is magnificently beautiful.

Water to Wine

The day rose to meet us with all of the perfection and possibilities of a humble life on earth. The swallows, which returned each year to the dozen or so houses Dale constructed for them, arrived once again, flitting and flirting above the meadow, scoping out the real estate. We sent the kids to the chicken coop to collect eggs for breakfast. *Real* Easter eggs! Over breakfast, we watched a small flock of Canada Geese touch down in the wet field and dance their mating rituals for us. Two male geese hissed, spat, and strutted for each other and for the attention and affection of a solitary female. We drank coffee on the deck as the sun climbed higher into the sky, pouring golden light into our day.

"What a beautiful day!" I must have said it ten times before 9:00 A.M. "We *have* to be outside today."

"We can make a fire and burn up a bunch of the wood scraps that are lying around," Dale offered.

"Perfect! We'll have a spring equinox/Easter fire ceremony!"

What a blessing it is to have some patch of land to care for on the day when spring arrives. The instinctual urge to interact with the spirit of the world is easily facilitated by the act of picking up sticks or cleaning up a garden patch. We were especially lucky to have sticks, branches, planks, two by fours, plywood, strapping, bits of posts and beams-- all manner of wood to collect. We piled it high and set it on fire, except for the choice sticks that had becomes swords for the elfin boys. They needed their swords to poke the fire, to raise as burning torches in celebration, to duel each other, and to protect the priestess (a.k.a. me) from the bad guys.

When the fire was sufficiently poked and the thrill of waving dangerously burning sticks in the air subsided, the boys and I agreed to go on an adventure in the woods. Safety officer Dale wanted to stay home and tend the fire, so Beau, Justin, and I set off across the meadow toward the lower beaver pond. Winter boots were the required footwear for traversing shaded sections of land where the slushy snow was still several inches deep, and for the sunny, bare, spots where the mud would suck an unsuspecting shoe right off the foot. The smell of death and birth mingled as our footsteps met the ground, driving upward an aromatic mixture of last season's dried hay and this year's tender green shoots. The first balmy breath of spring lifted our chins and opened our chests. I couldn't get enough, drinking the light nectar of life into lungs, ribs, and shoulders that had been contracted too long from the frigid winter assault.

"It's a beautiful day, isn't it, Mom?" Beau asked, leaning into my bliss. He always knows what I am thinking and how I am feeling.

"It *is* a beautiful day, Beau! It's a magical day! The land is welcoming us. Can you feel it? It's like the land is waking up because we live here now. We see the earth and she sees us."

"You're pretty happy today, aren't you, Mom?"

"Yes, I am, sweetie," I laughed. "Are you, too?"

"Yeah! I mean, we get to live here in such a

beautiful place. We're really lucky!"

"I know!"

As we approached the beaver dam, we were surrounded by the joyful symphony of water trickling through sticks, gurgling under thin layers of melting ice, and bubbling from underground springs.

Pure-of-heart Justin was captivated and immediately wanted to be one with the water. "There's water everywhere! Isn't it cool, Mom? You can hear it everywhere, but you can't really get to it. It's making me thirsty! Can we break the ice and drink from the stream?"

"Oh, no, honey, sometimes there are germs in streams that can really upset your stomach. Beavers or horses might live upstream and contaminate it. You shouldn't drink out of streams."

"Darn it! It's making me so thirsty."

"You can eat snow. It's probably not too dirty. Let's put our hands in the water, anyway."

I submerged my hands into the frosty stream where a hole had opened in the ice from the force of the rushing water below. In spontaneous ceremony, I touched my wet fingers to my forehead, then to my lips, and to my throat. Realizing that I couldn't leave out my heart, I dipped my fingers back in the stream and then reached down through layers of cotton, wool, and fleece to deposit a drop between my breasts. I finished the ritual by quickly blessing my solar plexus, belly, and root, although from the outside of my clothing, and then one last drop on the crown of my head.

"It's like baptism" I told the boys. "In the Christian

tradition newborn babies are baptized in a ceremony with water. Nowadays they just put a drop of water on their foreheads, but they used to dunk them all the way under the water. John the Baptist was a saint who used to baptize people in rivers. The ritual symbolized the washing away of sins of the past."

"What's a sin?" asked Beau.

"It's a wrongdoing, like hurting someone on purpose or lying or stealing. It depends on who you ask, really. The original meaning of the word sin comes from an archery term meaning to miss the mark. So I think of sin as more of like missing the connection with God and making bad decisions because your decisions are not coming from your spirit."

"But babies don't really do anything wrong, do they?"

"Well, no, but some people believe that everyone is born with what they call original sin, a sin that everyone is supposed to have because they are away from God. It has something to do with Adam and Eve. You know that story, where Adam and Eve were the first man and woman. They lived in the Garden of Eden, which was paradise, and they had everything that they needed to be happy. The story goes that God told them not to eat the fruit off of the tree of knowledge. A serpent, who is said to be the devil, talked Eve into eating the fruit, and she talked Adam into eating it. When God found out they had disobeyed him, he sent them out of the Garden of Eden as a punishment. Since we are all descendants of the first man and woman, we all carry that original sin. So they try to wash it away with water when babies are born."

"Damn women." Justin said in mock disgust, as he chomped on a snowball.

"Justin!" I admonished him for swearing as well as for blaming women, but we all giggled, because we all knew better.

"Did my sin get washed off?" asked Beau in a concerned voice.

"Well, I'm not sure I believe in original sin. Anyway, Beau, at least not in that way of looking at it, so I don't think you were guilty of anything when you were born. We did do a ceremony in the backyard when you were born, though, and we did use water to wash you clear of anything that didn't serve you as you came into your new life, and lavender oil to bless you and welcome your spirit. So, you're good."

"Okay, good."

"Anyway, if you have any concerns about that or anything else you want to wash away, you can do it now with *this* baptism. Put your hands right in the water and ask for any sin to be washed away. Spring is reborn at the equinox, Jesus is reborn at Easter, and we are constantly recreating ourselves every day."

I put my hands in the water again. There is only so much time to keep the attention of young boys, so I silently and expediently prayed for the release of anything that did not serve me in my new life. The boys put their hands in the water in turn. I didn't ask them what they were thinking or if they prayed. It seemed to be between each of us and spirit.

We continued across the stream at the outlet of the

dam and skirted the hemlock forest behind the beaver pond. Beau was in the lead as we passed a small stand of beech saplings on the left edge of the path.

"I have a runny nose, Mom." he said, and without a second thought, he ripped one of last season's dangling brown beech leaves from the undergrowth and swiped it under his nose.

I threw back my head in laughter.

"What, Mom?" Justin asked from behind me.

"I think the baptism worked!" I giggled. "Beau just blew his nose on a leaf like nature boy. He reached over and yanked off a dead leaf and went for it. He never does stuff like that! I love it. He was just all free and not worried about it being scratchy or gross or anything. We are all washed clean of our limitations, of our old thoughts, and of our fears on this watery day. I feel like we are living within a magical matrix today!"

We laughed and walked on, lifted by the essence of life rising out of the ground on the first spring day in Vermont. The sap was rising up from its winter home deep in the roots of the trees. Bulbs pushed upward, and grass unbent and stood erect. Everywhere we walked, the earth came to meet our senses. I was overflowing with the joy of love for life, for my boys, and for the woods. Love poured into me and flowed out of me. We circled around to the left, through the hemlocks, and followed the upper stream back to where it feeds into the top of the beaver pond. Standing before the half-frozen stream, we were once again met by the lilting melody of water, water everywhere. My eyes became fixed and glazed, my auditory channel tuned in, and I let the sounds of the water enter my ears and my mind with newness. Moving through the immediate and conditioned identification of the sound, I opened my innocent ears to the experience of listening to the water for long enough to hear something deeper. I met the essence and felt the energy of the water.

"The water is the blood of the earth, flowing everywhere, waking up from its deep freeze, flushing to the surface, and causing her cheeks to blush. These streams are like the blood vessels of the earth," I mused.

"Urgh! I just wish we could *drink* it!" Justin pleaded.

The melodic biblical line from the rock opera, *Jesus Christ Superstar*, dramatically sang out from my own circulatory system. "This is my blood you drink. This is my body you eat."

Images arose of Christ turning water into wine, and priests transforming wine into blood. I could see a silver chalice being ceremoniously removed from its holy little cloaked cubby where God transformed little glutinous wafers into the body of Christ when priests mumbled secret words.

What better symbol for the body and blood of Christ on this Easter day than the body and blood of the earth, awakened by the return of the sun? The atmosphere shifted almost imperceptibly, with a slight sharpening of purpose, and we slipped into sacred ceremony. We descended one notch deeper into divine awareness, and I knew the water had been rendered safe to drink. It had been transformed, as the priest transforms the wine into blood, by the prayers and intentions that brought us to this very moment.

"We *can* drink it!" I exclaimed. "Come on!"

As we knelt down next to the small rivulet flowing quickly from a spring to our right, I told the boys of the Christian ritual of the Eucharist. "You can catch some water in your cupped hands like this...or...I'm going to put my face right in it!" I slurped a little bit of the blood of the earth and held the boys steady as they bent over to put their mouths in the water, too.

"Now we need to eat the body of the earth," I continued. We foraged under dead grassy stalks and found some sweet, new sprouts. I pinched off three tiny pieces, and we each ate one, as I finished explaining that we were making our own rituals and honoring both Easter and the equinox. As we stood there in the silent grace of the day, two mallard ducks circled above us in their final approach for landing. We watched as they lowered their flaps and thrust out their landing gear, splashing down into the frigid pond. I opened my arms wide, breathed deep, and laughed at the perfection of life.

Justin smiled at me and chuckled, "Everything is really connecting for you today, isn't it, Mom?" As the witness, he drew my inner experiences out into the dimensions of daylight. Simply by acknowledging me, seeing me, communicating with me, he made it real.

"Yes it is, honey. It *really* is. We are living in Eden."

Epilogue

I am living, loving, and learning in Eden. I am practicing and teaching Zero Balancing in Eden. I am growing and flowering in Eden. I am well.

Wellness is a state of dynamic balance and requires conscious positive attention. It is a moment-by-moment series of decisions based on how much I allow my light to shine and how much I respect the awesome gift of my body. The autoimmune condition is just one of many possibilities that may or may not be expressed again. I am not afraid; I believe many of the cracks in my foundation, in which were sowed the seeds of disease, have been healed.

I remain willingly vigilant to my health, profoundly grateful for my gifts and blessings, awake to the lessons of life, and humbled by the fire of God's love that burns in my heart.

Appendix

Introduction to Zero Balancing

Waking to Eden is a story told, in part, through the lens of Zero Balancing (ZB). Zero Balancing is a mind-body therapy based on fundamental principles of nature. Practitioners of ZB touch the structure of the body while simultaneously touching the energy that animates it. As a bodywork practice, the results of consciously touching the interface of energy and structure in a body are strikingly profound. Equally profound is the insight that comes as practitioners of this healing art learn to touch energy in every other aspect of their lives. The principles of ZB are principles one can learn to live by and understand experiences through, resulting in an enhanced ability to sense a larger, and more integral reality, a world directed and created by energy exchange, by intention and attention. A world of order and purpose that exists simultaneously with global chaos.

A Zero Balancing session is done with the client lying on his or her back, fully clothed, on a treatment table. It is generally very relaxing and promotes an altered state of consciousness—a meditative state. Zero Balancing creates the opportunity for the release of outmoded patterns of thought, emotion, behavior, and physical posturing that keep one from being present, happy, and free. It does so by offering skilled touch to the deepest energy currents in the body—the energy in bone.

A ZB session is like a song played on the ivory keys of a human skeleton. The notes of the song are called *fulcrums*. Fulcrums are fields of tension (a gentle lift, stretch, twist, traction, etc) held at a point of stillness by the practitioner's hands. The relationship of the structure and the energy in the client reorganizes organically around this point of stillness, creating greater harmony in the body. Each session is a spontaneous symphony, and its signature is a composition of the essence of the client and how his or her body directs the placement of fulcrums based on accumulated physical, mental, emotional, or spiritual experiences. A full description of ZB can be found in *Inner Bridges* by Fritz Smith, MD[17] and *Zero Balancing, Touching the Energy of Bone*, by John Hamwee.[18]

Acknowledgments

Thank you to all who have shared in the long journey of bringing *Waking to Eden* to print. I am forever grateful to Julie Lineberger, faithful friend and writing partner. Thank you to Dr. Fritz Smith, Jim McCormick, Aminah Raheem Smith, Denise DiMauro, Mary Bove, Julian Jonas, Kayla Black, Lisa Berger, Elizabeth Gillespe, Barbara Levan, Kelly Salasin, Nancy Fullington, John Wimberley, Mary Beth McCarthy, Patti Bolagnani, JoEllen Kirsch, Eve Pearce, John Franklin, Joseph Cincotta, Gerry DeGray, Dano DeJong, Paul Lacinski and crew, the straw bale raising crew, and to the many readers of early versions of this manuscript for your support, expertise, and encouragement. To the staff at CreateSpace and to my editor, Lizzie Warren, much appreciation for how easy you made the process of publishing. Thanks to Jay Sullivan for your positive attitude and creative input in the design process. I sincerely appreciate the gift of the whole Morgan clan; love has always held my parents and eight siblings together in a profound bond of familial respect and admiration. Thank you, Eden, for your enduring presence. And mostly, thank you to my husband Dale and my sons Justin and Beau for your unending love and devotion.

Michele Morgan Doucette
April 4, 2010 (Easter Sunday)

Notes

[1] Ralph H. Blum, The Book of Runes, (New York: St. Martin's Press, 1993).

[2] Jaimie Sams and David Carson, Medicine Cards, (New York: St. Martin's Press, 1988).

[3] Genisis 1:2-3 (King James Verson).

[4] John Lennon and Paul McCartney, "Let it Be," *Let it Be*, 1970, Apple.

[5] Llewellyn Vaughn-Lee, Love is a Fire: The Sufi's Mystical Journey Home (Iverness, CA: The Golden Sufi Center,   2000).

[6] Emmylou Harris, "Cup of Kindness," *Stumble Into Grace*, 2003. Nonesuch Records.

[7] Paulo Coelho, The Alchemist, (Harper Torch, 1993, English translation).

[8] Joni Mitchell, "People's Parties," *Court and Spark*, 1974, Asylum.

[9] Robert Berkow, MD, editor, The Merck Manual of Diagnosis and Therapy, (New Jersey; Merck & Co., 1987).

[10] John O'Donahue, Anam Cara, audiotapes, (Boulder, CO, Sounds True Audio, 1996).

[11] The Byrds, "Turn, Turn, Turn (To everything there is a season)," *The Bitter and the Sweet*, 1962, Columbia.

[12] Robert Frost, "The Road Not Taken,: *Mountain Interval*, 1916.

[13] Mary Oliver, "The Summer Day," *New and Selected Poems*, (Boston, Beacon Press, 1992).

[14] Chris Bojalian, The Law of Similars, (New York, Random House, 1999).

[15] Garland E. Allen and Jeffrey J.W. Baker, Matter, Energy, and Life, (Reading, MA, Addison-Wesley, 1974).

[16] Mary Oliver, Wild Geese, *New and Selected Poems,* (Boston, Beacon Press, 1992).

[17] Fritz Frederick Smith, MD, Inner Bridges, (Atlanta, GA: Humanics New Age, 1986).

[18] John Hamwee, Zero Balancing: Touching the Energy of Bone, (Berkeley, CA: North Atlantic Books, 1999).

8923079R0

Made in the USA
Lexington, KY
13 March 2011